CEAC

The Indoor Epidemic

Praise for *The Indoor Epidemic*

In *The Indoor Epidemic*, Erik Shonstrom has reminded us of a basic truth that every traveler knows: learning occurs through experience, and the best experiences are those that happen when we venture out into the wide world."
—**Rolf Potts**, travel writer; author of *Vagabonding* and *Marco Polo Didn't Go There*

"In an era of standards-based education within a technology-obsessed culture, Shonstrom reminds us of the educational value that lies just beyond our classroom cages, in our own backyards and beyond. This rich research-based text will inspire any thoughtful educator or parent to empower young people to move and engage with the natural world around them."
—**Donna Terrell**, educator, Hillsborough County, Florida

"Inactivity is killing Americans. Humans weren't designed to sit at desks all day, and most of us started sitting at a desk in kindergarten. Shonstrom tackles not only the health consequences of our 'indoor epidemic,' but also its effects on our intellectual ability and spiritual well-being. He uses science, literature, and personal experience to argue that it all begins with an institutionalized educational system in need of change. I didn't agree with *every* opinion in the book, but *The Indoor Epidemic* definitely challenged my ideas of traditional education and made me rethink my beliefs."
—**Paul W. Slavik**, MD; hospitalist, internal medicine; assistant professor, University of Vermont College of Medicine

The Indoor Epidemic

How Parents, Teachers, and Kids Can Start an Outdoor Revolution

Erik Shonstrom

ROWMAN & LITTLEFIELD
Lanham · Boulder · New York · London

Published by Rowman & Littlefield
A wholly owned subsidiary of The Rowman & Littlefield Publishing Group, Inc.
4501 Forbes Boulevard, Suite 200, Lanham, Maryland 20706
www.rowman.com

Unit A, Whitacre Mews, 26–34 Stannary Street, London SE11 4AB

British Library Cataloguing in Publication Information Available

Library of Congress Cataloging-in-Publication Data Available

ISBN: 978-1-4758-2590-9 (cloth : alk. paper)
ISBN: 978-1-4758-2592-3 (electronic)

∞™ The paper used in this publication meets the minimum requirements of American National Standard for Information Sciences—Permanence of Paper for Printed Library Materials, ANSI/NISO Z39.48–1992.

Printed in the United States of America

This book is dedicated
with love and gratitude
to my kids, Vivien and Finn—
there's no mountain
I wouldn't climb for you.

Contents

Acknowledgments

Many thanks to Sarah Jubar, my editor at Rowman & Littlefield, who has supported and promoted the ideas in this book from the start. Thanks also to Meredith Nelson and Savitha Jayakumar for their hard work and attention to detail. My gratitude goes as well to Rashad Shabazz, John Bodley, Paul Jones, and Paul Andrews, folks who kindly gave me their time and expertise. I'm also indebted to Adam Rosenblatt, who elucidated children's right to play outside for me—thanks, Ad. I owe so much to the kind, patient folks who looked at chunks of this manuscript and were kind enough to talk about some of the ideas in these pages; gratitude is due to Brian Murphy, Jeff Rettew, and Dave Mills. I'm thankful to my family for the love they've shown me over the years, especially my father Mike Shonstrom, and stepmother, Amy, who've made the trek into northern Vermont time and again to show their support. My kids—Finn and Vivien—are the center of my world. I love you two past the horizon and back. Everything about my life that I'm grateful for eventually leads back to one person: my wife, Cindy. Whenever I am unsure of myself—in prose, profession, or personality—I know that she'll steer me straight, using the keen compass of her insight and the strength of her resolute honesty. Love you, Ghani.

Introduction

What happens to us when we step over the threshold and head into the outdoors? It's a question that's puzzled me my whole life. It's hard to deny that there is something that happens—a certain feeling, a particular frame of mind—which we encounter in the open air versus within four walls. As the English writer Geoff Dyer once noted: "I realised I could never experience a sense of spiritual arrival indoors."

Personally, I am intensely drawn to the outdoors—I feel a fierce urgency, every day, to *get out there*. As a teacher, I've projected this need onto my students, and as a result my teaching philosophy has largely been concerned with creating outdoor and experiential education events, trips, and journeys. This book, while written over the course of a year or two, represents a lifetime of embracing the outdoors as a multitude of metaphors in my life: freedom, escape, sustenance, learning, and, honestly, the very stuff of *meaning*. I've spent what is probably an unusual amount of time musing on the way in which we interact with the outdoors, and the way the outdoors enacts itself on us.

It's cliché, but I feel more alive outdoors. Once, when I crossed paths with a bear on a hike in the Sierras, I was filled with a sense of immense gratitude, awe, joy, and old-fashioned *happiness*. There was shorts-soiling fear too, but mostly I felt alive.

Often, when reading about the experience of the wilderness, writers try to find their way into some sense of transcendence. I certainly agree, but in my experience it is a peculiar type of transcendence. I certainly don't transcend my sorry, physical state; I feel every blister, scratch, and bug bite acutely. But in these moments, as I feel my body moving through space, I'm in direct communion with the very machinery of my being—lungs chuffing, heart thumping, muscles aching. My eyes wander, as does my mind. I am more in myself in these moments. If there is any transcendence, it is that I transcend the annoying realities of the institutionalized, codified, cataloged world.

In daily, civilized, indoor life, I become susceptible to petty jealousies, deceptive behavior, and anxiety-ridden rumination. But out there, I improve—I'm clearer, more focused in a cosmic sense by being less focused on the trivial. By any moral standard, or for that matter any calibration of personality and temperament, I'm a better person in nature.

In my limited experience, most students are, too. And as a teacher, that's what I have worked at to provide for my students: the chance to be better people. That's the opportunity I believe they have in the wild. Every kid deserves adventure, and the chance to be a hero.

That's a roundabout way of introducing part of the impetus behind this book. I think kids are their best selves when they're away from the atrophying succor of digital distraction. I think they're better away from the civilized world of adults that's at times fed by our own neurosis and insipid, fear and ego-based rationales and rules. Some of what we make children do in education, when looked at with clear eyes, is absurd, and may in fact inhibit learning. As Rousseau states in *Emile*, "I see nothing more stupid than these children who have been reasoned with so much."

We care about things that kids don't, but try to make them care, too, instead of trying to understand their values and wants. We've developed baseless means to assess competencies and calibrate student success through outdated and imprecise ideologies. We give minority students, children from challenged socioeconomic backgrounds, and diverse learners short shrift sometimes. Not all the time, but often enough that it makes sense to explore what the outdoors can do to mitigate some of these challenges.

Out there, in unstructured nature, kids have an even keel. They find autonomy. They have agency. They become themselves. Again, from Rousseau,

> Do you, then, want to cultivate your pupil's intelligence? Cultivate the strengths it ought to govern. Exercise his body continually; make him robust and healthy in order to make him wise and reasonable. Let him work, be active, run, yell, always be in motion. Let him be a man in his vigor, and soon he will be one in his reason.

Sounds like a solid pedagogy to me. Even if Rousseau himself was a pretty poor parent (he didn't raise his own kids—sort of abandoned them, actually) and we set aside the patriarchal tone of the writing.

But I'm no expert. Really, I'm an ideologically itinerant essayist who simply joneses for mountains more than anything else. Many of the ideas in this book rest upon research I've done in physiology, evolutionary biology, psychology, genetics, neuroscience, philosophy, history, literature, educational pedagogy, and race and gender studies. I've endeavored to be true to other's work as far as humanly possible. Whenever practical, I have attributed information to the original authors, interviews, or research I depended on. Any omissions, inaccuracy, or misinterpretations are my own fault.

Some of the names in this book have been changed out of respect for privacy. For more information on how the outdoors relates to learning and human development, a complete list of sources is available at the back of the book.

And now, let's go outside.

Chapter 1

The Curse of the Corner Office

We begin our day in a box. Not a nest or burrow—a box: the geometrical confines of our mattress. Our first act upon waking? Gazing into a small, pixelated box to await instruction. We box ourselves in the shower to slough off last night's dreams. Breakfast from a box. Heat it up in a box. Into our wheeled boxes, off to work to stare at another bright, absorbing box. Boxed lunch. After work, maybe pick up dinner in a box—head home to boxed entertainment. All indoors. Stuck in the box.

When asked to define ourselves on questionnaires, we are forced to box identities; male, female, white, black, biracial—no matter how limiting these boxes may be. We fill out forms online and check the box to signify our acceptance. It's ironic that we announce our boxed docility by clicking a button labeled, "submit."

Many of us, when we die, will be boxed up and filed away.

Our students and children are living lives that are more and more within boxes—both real and imagined. They play on the Xbox. They learn by filling in boxes. When we offer them the brief respite of outside playtime, what do they do? They scream, run—dash—out into the world. Gulp air in voracious breaths, talk loudly and with fervor, eyes sparkling with the sheer possibility the outside world offers. Then, in a flash, it's over. The bell rings.

Back in the box.

The most insidious barrier facing children's learning today is that schools are designed to make them sit, in chairs, at desks, for large chunks of time throughout the day. Students' bodies are forced into sedentary positions; their growing limbs, aching for movement, are all but bolted to plastic chairs that are bolted to desks that are, at times, bolted to the floor. Walking the halls of an elementary school, it's possible to hear the admonition "calm bodies!" from teachers, paraprofessionals, and parents as kids ramble down hallways—everyone seems intent on stifling movement from every quarter.

Even in physical education the curse of inertia has struck. When I was a reporter, I interviewed a physical education teacher as part of an assignment. I asked him if he loved what he did because he got to go outside and play—if he woke up happy every day because his very job description probably had the words "games" and "running" and "outdoors" in it. He stared at me incredulously and told me that going outside was something he tried to avoid. But, why? I stuttered. He told me that he couldn't get the kids to listen when they were outside, and the new standards for physical education (PE) required him to teach all kinds of stuff using worksheets and lesson plans. Going outside to play was now an obstacle to teaching PE, he said. He was one of the saddest men I've ever met.

The thing that's absolutely nuts is how pervasive this philosophy is—that learning works best, or can only occur, when students are sitting and still. Some schools are beginning to push back against this idea, introducing movement-oriented lessons and offering more dynamic activities that involve getting out chairs and walking around the room, but that sort of thinking dies out almost completely by middle school, and it's unlikely to discover movement-oriented learning (often called "kinesthetic learning") in most public high schools. In colleges, such as where I work, the expectation is often seventy-five-minute classes of sitting, listening, reading, and talking—but very little movement. In our own adult world this is even more pervasive. We all suffer through interminable days where we sit, and sit, and sit; it's brutal. It's torture.

In fact, the modern American workplace is perhaps even worse than schools—especially at meetings. When we're not staring at our little screens, we're called into a room to sit in a different chair and stare at a larger screen. Someone stands in front of the room, droning on, with a PowerPoint burning our retinas, or handing out sheets of paper with information that we couldn't possibly absorb since we're so physically sick due to the amount of inertia that's collected in our body. Our brains fall asleep, and our knees are bouncing to beat the band. Negative thoughts pool faster than the blood in our butts. And yet, we accept this—accept, for our kids and ourselves, this somnambulant experience that is the very essence of hypocrisy in terms of learning.

The fact is learning occurs most readily, authentically, and deeply when we're moving our bodies. When our bodies sit at rest, our brains take the day off, too.

Not only are children forced to sit for hours every day; they're caged indoors. They sit under the glare of fluorescent lights, and when they try to move—when their bodies revolt at what is the absolute antithesis of natural development for a young person—they get in trouble. They get labeled as disruptive. Teachers are unhappy because they have to be barking drill-instructors, begging, threatening, and manipulating students into sitting through a lesson; children are miserable because their very bodies are screaming to move and play and they're denied this basic right; parents are frustrated because Johnny and Jane keep getting in trouble for getting out of their chair. I am shocked every time I visit a school that the students don't toss their tablets or pens into the air and catapult out the windows, fleeing this barbaric denial of their right to physically move on a regular basis throughout the day.

At the core of this snarled web is a basic misconception: that learning is inseparable from quiet, focused, still, and seated study. How can children possibly learn while running about, free, and in the open air? How could they remember anything that happened, anything they were told? As the layers are peeled back, however, it becomes clear that learning is not something that occurs *separately* from movement, or even that *can* occur at times during physical movement. When we dig deep into our evolutionary, psychological, and neurological makeup, we discover that learning *is* movement. They are inseparable, and one in the same.

What these sacks of bone and muscle and blood we call bodies are good for—and why that matters in terms of learning—is part of the puzzle, as are the psychology of being indoors, infant development, and a wide array of other factors, including emerging research in embodied cognition studies. But to begin to understand why having children move their bodies—and especially move their bodies outdoors—is inseparable from learning, we need to explore what, exactly, our bodies evolved to do. Understanding our physical history as a species is the first step in unlocking the door and getting back outdoors to learn.

THE FLAMINGO'S BEAK

In the book *The Flamingo's Smile*, the late evolutionary biologist Stephen Jay Gould wrote about the morphology of the flamingo's big, hooked schnoz and offered up some clues as to the relationship between the shape of bodies and body parts in nature and the behavior of animals.

A classic example of this kind of adaptation is the giraffe. The giraffe—at once aristocratically elegant and adolescently gawky—evolved a long neck because it was an advantage. Being able to eat leaves way up high that other animals can't reach is an adaptive strategy—it works. What Gould and many biologists question is how the *shape* of an animal's body affects behavior, and vice versa. This is especially true when a species enters a new ecosystem—how will its behavior and morphological characteristics play out in terms of reproductive success?

A pertinent example here is that of the rock dove. In the wild, these birds once nested primarily on sea cliffs and mountainsides. They evolved broad, powerful wings to execute smart, sharp turns in the vertiginous landscapes where they nested and lived; a compact, glossy body; and an ability to exploit their environment by being ecumenical eaters. Now, of course, we call them "rats with wings," and the common street pigeon is found in the tens of millions in thousands of cities around the world. Originally domesticated and then gone feral, this once-wild bird has been able to capitalize on its preference for rocky cliff sites for nests and use the buildings that line 5th Avenue in Manhattan just as well.

Not every animal fares as well, however, with new or changing ecosystems. One of the most familiar examples, of course, is the dodo bird, a now-extinct species of large flightless bird that once inhabited the island of Mauritius in the Indian Ocean. The introduction of a couple of ravenous species (humans, rats, dogs, and pigs) wiped out the poor dodo in the seventeenth century. While some species like rats, pigeons, and seagulls are able to exploit multiple habitats, others don't do as well. Much of this has to do with morphology.

Humans are another example of a species that has proved very successful at exploiting multiple ecosystems and environments, from deserts to rainforests to the food court at the mall. Looking backward, a fair question seems to be what, exactly, our bodies evolved to do.

For instance, our brachiating cousins, the gibbons, are well designed to swing through tropical canopies, but less adept at walking along the ground. A detailed analysis of our own physiology is necessary to understand what we evolved to do, in what kind of environment, and for what purpose. This, in turn, will help us understand why—despite the fact that we love our new ergonomic chair with the breathable mesh back and our large format computer monitor—being indoors sitting down all day may be at odds with a few million years of evolution.

As far as body size goes, humans are pretty average. The average weight of all terrestrial mammals—including elephants, hippos, and tapirs but also chipmunks, pygmy shrews, and bats—is around 100 pounds. Nowadays, we're a bit heavier than that on average. The American body is the biggest in the world, averaging about 175 pounds. But for most of our evolutionary history, 100 pounds would've been about right. We are a mid-sized mammal. As Stephen Jay Gould noted, bodies and behavior go hand in hand. Aardvarks grow big claws and long tongues because they eat termites; they have to dig open cement-hard termite mounds and slurp up all the little insects. Which brings us to our central question: what, exactly, are humans built to do?

BUILT TO MOVE

At first glance, not much. Comparatively speaking, humans are not strong. Humans' closest evolutionary cousins—bonobos and chimpanzees—are twice as strong, according to recent findings published by the *Proceedings of the Royal Society B: Biological Sciences*. Humans are sorely lacking in the beak, antler, tooth, and claw department. People aren't particularly fast, and most similarly sized mammals like antelopes, wolves, leopards, and springboks could beat humans in a race easily. The fastest human at the time of this writing, the Jamaican Olympian Usain Bolt, tops out at a bit shy of twenty-eight miles per hour, a speed easily beaten by most terrestrial mammals—even kangaroos can hop at over forty miles per hour. But if there's one thing humans do well as a species, it's ramble across large swaths of terrain.

Human beings are one of the animal kingdom's great wanderers and explorers.

With long legs, hairless bodies that sweat and effectively discharge heat, and the ability to breath off-sync with movements (unlike many galloping animals, who have to breathe in time with the cadence of their legs due to their internal organs' morphology), hominids are quite literally built to cross rugged landscapes in search of food, water, and new resources.

Harvard anthropology professor Daniel Lieberman is well known in evolutionary biology circles as the creator and most vocal proponent of the "persistence hunter" theory. This idea suggests that humans evolved a number of remarkable adaptations to chase prey in the heat of the day. Hairless bodies that sweat very effectively, breathing through noses and mouths to get lots of oxygen and expel heat, springy tendons in long legs, and large brains allowed early humans to trot after game as it tired out in the hot African sun. While humans may not be particularly fast and strong, it turns out that among the animal kingdom they're up there with the best of them endurance-wise, able to cover large distances at a steady pace almost as well as horses and dogs.

With an unrivaled ability to cross vast terrain at a decent clip, bipedal hominids are built to be explorers. Add hands with incredibly fine motor control that can pick up and examine all kinds of objects, and a large brain that is exceedingly curious about its environment, and the sum is a rambling, wandering species that can jog, climb, and investigate the world around it with relative ease. And, if Lieberman's theory is correct, it was this morphology that allowed humans to hunt game that otherwise would not have been accessible as a food source—a vital adaptation that may have played a major role in the human species' success as it spread across the globe out of Africa.

We're built to move. Everything about our bodies—the way we have rubbery ligaments in our necks to keep our heads steady when we run; the way our eyes can shift their focus from the horizon to the ground in front of our feet in a split second; and the way our arms swing and help us keep balance—it's all been designed by evolution to help us move over the terrain.

And yet, we force our students to sit, inside, in chairs, rather than capitalize on their evolutionary advantages. It's like asking a lion to sit in an office chair and color-code a spreadsheet. It's ridiculous. We're not built to sit still.

The connection between learning and our evolutionary origins as landscape traversing forager/hunters may not at first seem all that clear. However, there has been some interesting research into how those hunts worked—how human's Paleolithic ancestors jogged along after prey over miles and miles—and the impact it had on the development of our cognition, even our imagination.

How does the ability to run long distances in the prehistoric past have any bearing on the ability to learn? The first place to look for that answer is the brain itself. Endurance running is a brain booster—it pumps up various regions of the brain and increases the number of synapses. Not only that, but navigating across the landscape—free-ranging—and having to remember where food, water, shelter, and predators are located is all part of spatial learning.

Spatial learning is a vital component of what makes humans so adept at understanding patterns and systems like trigonometry and fantasy football drafts. It has a direct effect on the hippocampus, a small part of the brain tucked under the big cauliflower-looking part that helps store memories and make new ones. In fact, studies have increased the size of the hippocampus in rats by up to 30 percent simply by giving them environments they had to explore, navigate, and remember.

In a paper published in *Frontiers in Neuroscience* in 2014, researcher Mark Mattson states: "Studies of rodents, monkeys, and humans have shown that running can increase the size of several different brain regions including the hippocampus and midbrain." Mattson's study goes on to explain why, exactly, this has a bearing on how humans learn as a species:

> The ability of running to improve pattern processing is evolutionarily conserved, as demonstrated in experiments with rats and mice showing that running enhances hippocampus-dependent spatial pattern separation. In humans, running improves mood and enhances cognitive and sensory—motor capabilities.

It would be overly simplistic to say that running across the landscape trying to tire out a wildebeest is going to get a kid into Harvard, but on a purely neurological level it seems clear that there is a definite connection between a healthy brain and movement.

It makes sense as an evolutionary adaptation. Individuals who covered lots of ground, remembered where the fruit was ripening, were successful at chasing down animals for food, and knew the best shelter in their territory would have a distinct advantage and pass those skills through their genes to their offspring. It also makes sense that the individuals who could learn during this process would have the benefit of not just keeping track of existing resources but figuring out how to exploit new ones. This ability to predict and respond to environmental stimuli based on information gained by moving about is how spatial learning provides the template for more advanced forms of learning and cognition.

If spatial learning is the process where animals, including humans, collect and interpret information about their environment that guides their movements and aids them in remembering important information about their surroundings, a probable antecedent of this ability is the application of the same memory oriented skills to thinking that is more abstract in nature such as symbolism. It's the basic template, cognition-wise, for understanding systems, patterns, and repetition. It could be argued it's the basis of learning.

What happens when children are denied the chance to develop this crucial ability? What happens when their brains don't get to grow as they navigate the outdoors? We may be starting to see the results in the form of sharply spiking rates of depression, learning disorders like attention deficit hyperactivity disorder (ADHD), and obesity. The way spatial learning works—and its benefits for other kinds of learning—seems to be central to how humans' cognitive abilities evolved. But for now, let's get back inside the classroom and check out what students are doing, if they're *not* learning outside.

15,000 HOURS

Search your memory. There were times when you probably liked school. Some gifted teacher was talking or leading you through an activity, and you felt that heady spark of learning—the excitement that comes with gaining new information or skills. Or maybe you remember working on a really interesting project—a poster that documented the civil rights movement, or a model of an Algonquin longhouse. Those moments were great, inspirational, and, if we are honest, few and far between. What did we do with the bulk of our time? What about all those hours, all those days, that we don't remember, that don't exist in our brain's files?

If school takes up about 7 hours a day, and a student goes to school for 180 days each year, that totals well over 15,000 hours of school time by high school graduation, not counting kindergarten. 15,000 hours. That's a *huge* amount of time—massive, really. It's the equivalent of more than 600 days of school. That's over a year and a half of nothing but being in the classroom! What were we doing during all that time, as our bodies grew, as our concept of "self" began to flower, as we negotiated relationships, developed passions, and began to explore the world around us and within us?

The answer, unfortunately, is sad: we were sitting on our asses. A lot.

Sitting in chairs is a relatively recent phenomenon, at least as far as our evolutionary history is concerned. In fact, use of chairs for daily sitting didn't really reach most of the people on the planet until the sixteenth century. Prior to that, chairs were usually owned by aristocracy and were often more symbols of power than utilitarian items. Normal folks sat on chests, stools, or, more commonly, the ground.

The tradition of reserving chairs for those in control has carried on to the current day. It's no coincidence that the authority figures in committees are called "chairs" and that an endowed teaching position at a college is often called a "chair," and that the positions within the British House of Commons are called "chairs." Chairs not only have a history of representing authoritarian rule, hierarchies, and aristocracy; they're crazy bad for your body.

The very earliest evidence of chairs is from around the Egyptian dynasties, roughly 5,000 to 6,000 years ago. But prior to that—for the period that spans most of our history as evolutionary modern humans—the primary means of resting when not sleeping was squatting. Humans hunkered down, knees splayed, feet planted, and did whatever they needed to do; made fires, carved some wood, admired the handiwork on a new atlatl. For a perfect tutorial in how to squat, just swing by the closest daycare or kindergarten and watch the children playing outside. Kids—especially toddlers and young children—are champion squatters, happily spending most of their days alternating between careening about bipedally, crawling through the mud and bushes, or hunkering down in a squat to examine bugs and dig in the dirt.

WHAT IF WE ALL POPPED A SQUAT?

Now, of course, except for "circle time," we make kids sit in chairs. As adults, we also sit in chairs and even instruct children in the "correct" way of sitting; feet on the floor, butt scooched back, head and neck raised, back straight. The problem is that even with this very stuffy advice, sitting in a chair is just about the worst thing you can do to a kid—or yourself. Here's what "The Health Hazards of Sitting" from the *Washington Post* tells us happens when you sit and surreptitiously watch all those Key and Peele videos all day at your desk:

- Heart Disease: when you're not moving, your body is storing up all the fatty acids that would usually be burned by muscles and those nice artery-cloggers are ending up in your heart.
- Pancreas: your pancreas pumps out insulin to carry glucose to muscles. However, when muscles are idle, your body overproduces insulin because

non-active muscles don't respond as well to insulin uptake, which can lead to diabetes.

- Cancer: Yep, the big C. Primarily colon, breast, and endometrial kinds. Movement boosts natural antioxidants that fight cancer. Studies have linked long sitting to the development of various cancer cells.
- Abs, Hips, and Butt: This one is no surprise: by sitting all day these three areas of our body, which we've been socially conditioned to be horrified by if they're not taut and lean, slump into fat and disuse. Aside from the totally imaginary aesthetic principle we attach to these body parts, they're also vital for posture and general overall health.
- Circulation: deep vein thrombosis, varicose veins, and swollen ankles, anyone? Sitting gives 'em to you.
- Back, neck, and brain: the posture we assume while sitting is unnatural for our spine, and usually the cant of our head as we stare at the screen is bad for our neck. Add to that the fact that lack of movement and exercise makes our brain cloudy, and it's hardly a recipe for genius—or health.

Schools force children to sit in desks for extended periods, every day, despite the fact that it's clear that it's bad for them. Not only is the research conclusive; intuitively we know sitting is damaging our bodies.

For the sake of argument, let's just say that we relied on the old squatting position for activities that required students to be still. What would be the advantages?

Well, squatting is the default resting position for most of the world, and for most of our human history; we're built for it (for a humorous look at the advantages of squatting, watch the YouTube music video called "The Squat Song"). The problem is that shortly after our toddler years, we start getting forced into chairs. Bad backs, bad health, and all kinds of unfortunate circumstances result.

But squatting is not only beneficial—it's free and you can do it everywhere. The benefits for our students' bodies would be enormous: backs would get stretched, particularly the lower back, where much of the damage from sitting occurs. It's good for digestion (and, ahem, elimination). It reduces expenditures—no need to buy that Eames chair for three grand. For those of you thinking that you couldn't possibly function at your high-stress, screen-focused job, know that as I type these words I'm squatting on my kitchen floor, with my laptop on a simple wooden box in front of me. My back is stretched, my hips flexible, and I'm close to snacks. Win–win.

So the fact that we're terrain exploring animals has helped us grow big brains, and yet within the place where in the modern world we're supposed to grow our brain—school—movement is restricted. And not only is movement restricted, but it's replaced by sitting in chairs, which is bad for our bodies, rather than adopting a more natural position. But there's something much deeper here that is disturbing about the fact that school happens mostly indoors and sitting down; it may be killing our imagination.

TRACKING COGNITION

One of the theories proposed by anthropologists is that traversing the landscape—scouring the terrain for new resources or signs of potential prey or chasing down that prey—is a fundamental step in the development of cognition in *Homo sapiens*. According to work done by Louis Liebenberg, a South African scientist whose research has focused on the connections between the tracking activities of hunter-gatherers and the development of cognition, tracking may have been a first, important step in the fostering of the human species' capacity for an analytic, scientific mindset.

Liebenberg writes: "From an evolutionary point of view, the origin of the creative scientific imagination due to natural selection *by* nature may explain why it is so successful *in* nature." Liebenberg has studied the tracking of various tribes of nomadic hunter-gatherers in South Africa including the !Xo and others. His work documents the amazingly complicated process that goes into tracking animals through the arid South African bush.

Recognizing spoor; identifying tracks; reading the landscape; understanding the capacities, life histories, endurance, and feeding habits of prey animals—all this was used by nomadic trackers to create a narrative of the animals they were hunting. What are their evasive maneuvers; do they flee, burrow into the ground, or climb a tree? Turn and fight? There's little doubt that reading meaning into the text of nature is a complicated, multifaceted task that goes way beyond hurling a spear at a passing antelope and hoping for the best. If there are any lingering doubts, think you can head into the wilderness and try to feed yourself and your kin without a Dunkin Donuts nearby? Me neither.

The conceptual strands that connect what may be the earliest science—tracking animals for food—and the experience provided for children in schools are clear. And while the strands may appear at first to be a delicate bricolage of theory and conjecture, there's enough to suggest some interesting correlations between being outside, navigating unstructured outdoor landscapes and the development of cognition, and even, maybe, imagination.

What better way to introduce children to science, to conjecture and hypothesis, to research and study, than out in the woods, trying to read animal sign? That dug up a piece of turf there—is there an acorn buried underneath? Who buried it? Watching the squirrels, we see them leap their arcs from branch to ground and deposit their winter's cache. These holes drilled in a dead tree—what kind of bird did this work? Or was it something else? We hear hammering deep in the woods, and watch intently as northern flickers perch there, busily harvesting grubs from beneath the bark of withered pine. Through these adventures, we develop an appreciation for observation, testing, evidence, and proof—the cornerstones of science and analytic thinking.

I'm lucky to live in Vermont, where I can take my son hiking in the Green Mountains, or, if I'm willing to take the ferry across the slate gray waters of Lake Champlain, we can climb the Adirondack High Peaks. On these hikes, I'm always struck by my son Finn's incessant curiosity—his questions, his chatter. While we may walk nine, ten, even twelve hours through the day, he never seems particularly bored. Rather, something about the act of moving through the landscape both satiates and inspires his thoughtfulness—most of the time he is engaged in the world around him in a direct, kinesthetic way and at the same time existing in the world that resides deep in his imagination.

HYENA PACKS AND TASTY TUBERS

This act of moving through the woods, or the savannah, or any natural environment, may have played a major role in the development of how we negotiate both the world around us and symbolic systems like language. Thomas Wynn is an anthropologist at the University of Colorado in Colorado Springs. Some of his work has focused on human evolution and the development of our spatial abilities. Wynn believes that the development of "working memory" may have been "pivotal" in human evolution.

Working memory is how our mind holds onto, remembers, and processes information we gather from our environment but also other "neural sources" like long-term memory. Wynn believes that working memory underpins much of what we now refer to as "executive functions" in the brain, thus suggesting that understanding the development of working memory from an evolutionary perspective can help us see what role it plays in the fostering of higher levels of thought.

Remembering where the hyena pack hangs out, which fruit tree is ripening, and where the tasty tubers are in your landscape requires a dense web of memory and visuospatial image processing—basically, is that baobab tree over there the one closest to the spring, or is it *that* one over there? The ability to do this required our earliest ancestors to remember the shape and look of specific landscape features, and attach significance to them. We also had to gauge season, as we didn't want to travel to the vernal pool in the dry season when it was just a dusty depression in the ground. All of this involves memory, planning, calculation, and premeditation—the very stuff that makes up intellectual thought. And the environment where this occurs most readily is in the outdoors.

Humans have these abilities—innately. These abilities evolved in conjunction with the navigation and exploration of environment. However, the question remains whether or not it's detrimental to neglect engaging in those lower order skills—negotiating the unstructured landscape—before moving on to more relevant cognitive tasks such as reading the instructions for a shelving unit from IKEA. In looking at children, some of the evidence seems to suggest that denying them the experience of navigating the natural world could lead to a disorientation more profound than not knowing where to find the latrine on a camping trip. By not exercising these foundational exploratory experiences, schools could be isolating children from the very act of reengaging their most basic intellectual skills.

LANDSCAPE AND LEARNING

Bruce Chatwin's book *Songlines* tells the stories of the peripatetic writer's adventures down under. Chatwin, a late twentieth-century British author who danced the line between fact and fiction in his work, states that he's headed to Australia to understand more about the songlines. Songlines are Aboriginal paths, or tracks, across the vast reaches of Australia that, according to Aboriginal beliefs, were created by the original "creator beings" at the beginning of the world. Chatwin describes them thus: "Aboriginal Creation myths tell of the legendary totemic beings who had wandered over the continent in the Dreamtime, singing out the name of everything that crossed their path—birds, animals, plants, rocks, waterholes—and so singing the world into existence."

Chatwin's book (call it a novel or travelogue) bears on the conversation about being outside, rambling around the countryside for two reasons. First, his book highlights the way the earliest modern humans developed a symbolic mythology—the beginning of story, narrative, and complex imaginary beliefs—which could be considered the first body of intellectual knowledge in human history. The fact that this act was intimately tied to walking the landscape is vital. Second, Chatwin's book helps define what it is, exactly, about this act of walking through the landscape that is tied to learning.

Because Australia was one of the last places in modern history to be colonized by the western world, it is a useful place to examine the lives and beliefs of peoples who lived outside of the influence of industry, agriculture, centralized economy, and large-scale belief systems like Christianity and capitalism. One of the questions that puzzles anthropologists is when, exactly, did our big brains start developing the ability for abstract thought, for cognition, for planning and imagination? Due to the late contact with Europeans, the records of Aboriginal culture (before it was systematically destroyed by colonial powers) are one of the best avenues into this mystery.

Aborigines lived with no maps, books, or institutionalized knowledge about their world. And yet they navigated through the parched landscape of Australia by these songlines. A *basic* definition of the songlines is that the original creator beings sang their way across the world and passed those songs down to their "clans" or groups as a way of telling stories about the landscape, explaining natural features, and intimately tying the lives of the people of Australia to the very earth and its shapes. For instance, Australian Aborigines might sing of "possum dreaming" or "emu dreaming" as they walked the landscape. It was a means of navigation as well as a mythology—both a practical tool and the basis of their cultural understanding.

A pile of rocks could be "two koalas sleeping," for instance, and the song would tell the story of why they slept there. If this is true, then the very earliest stirrings of abstract thought—of story, legend, symbolism, and narrative—were wrought by the act of crossing the landscape. Therefore, the development of imagination happened on foot, moving through the world at walking speed.

The connection with learning requires some excavation and a bit of speculation, but it seems clear that the development of humans' big brains (with their ability to plan bridal showers, navigate Walmart, and write sonnets) came about in conjunction with the species' nomadic wanderings. It may not be a question of what came first. Perhaps they were concurrent. And if this is true, then the idea of teaching children while they're sitting down, fastened to a chair, is ludicrous. It was the German philosopher Johann Georg Hamann who wrote, "When I rest my feet my mind also ceases to function."

This concept is solidly backed up by science. Brains respond positively to exercise, to experience. And by respond what is meant is that they develop new synaptic connections; for example, the hippocampus responds by increasing its size. Exercise increases all sorts of positive mechanisms in human bodies, from strengthening the immune system to benefiting our respiratory functions. Our evolutionary history suggests that humans quite literally walked their way into the modern ability to think abstractly. As philosopher Søren Kierkegaard wrote, "I have walked myself into my best thoughts."

Chatwin's book is fantastic, and in the final pages he begins to unravel his big idea, one that is both startlingly radical and completely plausible. Whenever I read it, I think of my son when he was a toddler, and how he'd walk out into the field and forests, and turn around and gaze back at me, the world spinning around him as he breathed and lived and took it all in during that moment—alive and aware of his own body, his own perception—moving through the world. It also makes me wonder about the role the outdoors could have in the work we do in education to help our students along the path of their development—social, emotional, and intellectual. Chatwin writes:

> And here I must take a leap into faith: into regions I would not expect anyone to follow. I have a vision of the Songlines stretching across the continents and ages; that wherever men have trodden they have left a trail of song (of which we may, now and then, catch an echo); and that these trails must reach back, in time and space, to an isolated pocket in the African savannah, where the First Man opening his mouth in defiance of the terrors that surrounded him, shouted the opening stanza of the World Song, "I AM!"

Chapter 2

Paleoeducation

The function of school is hotly debated. Indeed, it could be said that school has many purposes, depending on who you ask. Some claim the function of school is to create "good citizens," while others say it is to train the future workforce. And while we can sit around and argue endlessly about all the different attributes and qualities and skills we hope education imbues in our students, we can all agree on a simple fact: school should make kids smarter.

But what does it mean to be smart? My $249 Google Chromebook is far smarter than I on an informational basis. Click a few buttons on it and it can answer any question I can possibly think to ask. With this device and an Internet connection, I have an almost infinite amount of information at my fingertips. While we all know that the processing and memorization of information is a part of learning, we also recognize that no matter how much data an individual possesses, it doesn't necessarily make that person smart. For instance, there are people who can recite pi to the 1000th digit, but that's not a particularly *useful* skill unless you're a mathematician. It won't help you get a job in most places, handle the complexities of modern romance in the Tinder generation, or keep track of all the intrigue on Game of Thrones.

It's not just skills that make us smarter, either. Let's say you develop—over years of careful diligent training—the ability to drive a golf ball and drop if perfectly into the cup on the green for a hole-in-one from 300 yards away every single time without fail. While an admirable and extremely rare and complicated skill, it's not going to—in and of itself—make you smarter. But just as my Chromebook is designed to be incredibly smart from an informational and computational perspective, it is also conceivable that a few scientists from Pasadena's Jet Propulsion Laboratory could design a machine that swings a golf club and has equal, or more likely greater, accuracy than you at driving a ball 300 yards on the links. High-level aptitude in incredibly narrow skill sets are not, in and of themselves, evidence of being "smart," either.

So if being smart isn't only the memorization of information, nor is it only the perfect execution of a particular skill set, than what is it? We can all agree that at least *part* of the definition of what it means to be "smart" includes the memorization of information and the execution of specific skills, but that's not everything involved with smartness—when we meet someone smart, or imagine ourselves gaining that quality, there is an associated list of abilities, skills, comprehensions, and perceptions. The individuals we consider smart have a large number of facets to their intellect.

Researchers who study intelligence usually define smartness as having critical, analytical, or problem-solving capabilities. My Chromebook can tell you the population of Copenhagen, but if my kitchen sink drips, the damn computer just sits there mute while my water bill goes through the roof. It can't actually *fix* anything. The clock ticking in my living room keeps precise, exact time of every second, minute, and hour that passes, but when my son comes home feeling crushed because he got yelled at by a teacher at school, my clock is poorly designed to console him and talk him through how to deal with getting in trouble and how to avoid it in the future. Both of these problems—one a physical issue that requires all kinds of tools, learning, trial-and-error, analysis, foresight, and experience; and the other that involves interpersonal empathy and compassion—are the sorts of challenges that require some degree of intelligence, but intelligence of a specific sort. They require abstract thought.

Stripping school down to its essential functions, this is what we're trying to do: *increase our students' capacity for abstract thinking.* Understanding the biology of abstract thought is key, then, if we are to explicate how to best engender it in our students, and how to work as educators to maximize our students' potential.

TIGER SHARK PERISTALSIS

Although reality television like the *Real Housewives* series offers convincing evidence to the contrary, we're one of the smartest species on the planet. But while our abstract thinking is remarkable, it's not wholly out of step with the rest of the creatures on earth. In short: we're not special.

Other animals such as chimpanzees, certain bird species, and dolphins have exhibited incredible problem-solving skills and abilities—arguably the real-world manifestation of abstract thinking. Not only that, but they demonstrate this ability in replicating human success in human-designed tasks. If the roles were reversed, and humans had to complete the kind of challenges faced in the animal world, I doubt any of us could come close to the kind of problem-solving capabilities of dolphins: dodging sharks, catching fish in our mouths, and using clicks and whistles to navigate the dark seas. We wouldn't last very long until we ended up enjoying the digestive massage of peristalsis in a tiger shark's intestine.

Abstract thought is best defined as the ability to analyze a situation, predict outcomes, weigh various approaches to problem solving, attach meaning to disparate events to understand some overarching narrative of action, and balance sensory perception, cognition, and action in such a way as to produce favorable results. The way this sort of thinking exists both in the brain and in the body is known as embodied cognition, a rapidly developing school of thought that posits that cognition is a whole body experience, not just a detached, intellectual event.

One of the easiest ways to understand abstract thought is to think about how we prepare for a job interview. We use our imagination to project ourselves into the future, envision ourselves cleverly answering questions. We anticipate those questions and develop appropriate responses, and even plan what to wear to appear more stylish and put together than we actually are. We may even fabricate alternate realities—otherwise known as lies—to trick our interlocutors into thinking we're smarter and more qualified than we actually are.

At its most high functioning, abstract thought allows us to create symbols, envision imaginary worlds we may go to when we die, and create an entirely imaginary value system around little slips of green paper with pictures of long-dead presidents on them.

The biological roots of abstract thought are generally thought to have taken hold around the times our brains got big. The part of our brain designed for this kind of thinking is the prefrontal cortex. Between about 500,000 and 50,000 years ago, humans evolved their big brains to handle the challenges represented by the hunter-gatherer-forager existence on the savannahs of Africa. This endocranial expansion happened before language, agriculture, cities, and writing. One way to look at it is to say that the ability to speak and write and grow yams didn't make our brains big; we had big brains already that made language and alphabets and farming an option.

Gerald Crabtree is a researcher and professor from Stanford who argues that the intellectual abilities of modern humans are genetically fragile and could possibly decline. The whys and wherefores of this are a complicated mix of evolutionary theory and genetics, but understanding the role genes play in our intelligence as a species is helpful if as educators we are to think about schools and the outdoors in a way that encompasses a tacit understanding of our evolutionary history and its repercussions. This isn't to say that we need our students chasing down gazelles and eating raw meat, squatting naked in the bush, but if, as Crabtree argues, our intellectual and emotional abilities are waning, it makes sense as educators to understand why.

A quick note here: the time spans we're talking about are *huge*—thousands of years long. The research presented here covers a vast amount of time. This stuff doesn't happen overnight. The deterioration of intellect according to Crabtree's work—in terms of genetics—takes thousands of years to enact itself.

Professor Crabtree's theory rests upon an understanding of a couple of ideas central to evolution: the pressures exerted by natural selection, genetic adaptation, the way genes mutate, and the diversity of genes involved in our intellectual abilities.

Many of our daily rituals; reading the morning news, writing a get-well card for a friend, toasting a bagel and spreading cream cheese on it, and helping our colleagues decipher some weird new draconian workplace policy involving the copier are quite complex and require a large number of genes to complete. For instance, yeast, which researchers often use in genetic studies because it replicates so quickly and has a relatively small number of genes (the yeast genome has about 5,300 genes, humans have about 20,000, give or take a few thousand), while still containing a great deal of genes, cannot back the car out of the driveway while scolding a toddler for spilling juice all over her car seat. Take that, yeast!

Warning: numbers approaching. Proceed with caution.

Crabtree offers us this analysis to help us understand how there's a fair number of genes involved in human intelligence and why that makes our intellect surprisingly fragile in terms of genetic mutation. Men have only one X chromosome, making it a good place to start thinking about how all this works. According to one particular study, on male X chromosomes there are a total of 818 X chromosome protein-coding genes, of a total of 19,586 genes. Studies of intellectual deficiencies that arise from the X chromosome are called X-linked intellectual deficiency (XLID). Of those 818 protein-coding genes on the human X chromosome, 215 give rise to XLID when mutated. Crabtree posits that "this line of evidence indicates that about ¼ of genes on the human X chromosome are needed for full intellectual and emotional function."

Crabtree hedges his bet and suggests that even if we use a "more conservative estimate of about 10% of the genes" that it still represents a large fraction of our total genetic package that genetically determines intellectual functioning. A key part of this theory is that genes don't necessarily function like a network, but more like old-school Christmas lights; if one bulb burns out, the rest of the chain doesn't work. Or, as Crabtree puts it, "failure of any one of the links gives rise to deficiency."

Here's where the numbers come in and we get to the heart of the argument. Basically, Crabtree is arguing that the proper functioning of between 2,000 and 5,000 genes is required for our ability to be intelligent, emotionally competent individuals. Individual protein-coding genes experience "deleterious mutations" (good name for a band) about once every 100,000 generations. After a complicated number of calculations, this pans out as follows:

> If indeed 2,000 to 5,000 genes are necessary for our intellectual and emotional stability than about one in 20 to 50 should suffer a new mutation affecting intellectual function. Another way to state the same information is that every twenty to fifty generations we should sustain a deleterious mutation. Within 3,000 years or about 120 generations we have all very likely sustained two or more mutations harmful to our intellectual or emotional stability.

This boils down to a basic idea: the pressure exerted by natural selection must be very high to keep up the "fitness" of our genetically inheritable intelligence traits because the large number of genes involved in intelligence and emotional fitness make mutations with negative results all the more probable. In honor of Professor Crabtree himself, think of your smart-genes this way: if you have a great big crate of apples and there's a bunch that are mushy and rotten, it's likely the rot will spread and ruin the whole crate. To use Crabtree's words: "The consequence is that selective pressure must be higher to maintain neurologic traits in general."

Now, finally, we can circle back to the central question underpinning this little detour: What is it about our Paleolithic, evolutionary origins that gave rise to our intelligence? Why is that very adaptive intelligence under siege and facing possible decay? And what does this have to do with getting kids outdoors more often?

HUNTER-GATHERER GENIUSES

The first part of the answer is that the selective process (i.e., the environmental forces that spurred adaptation in our prehistoric ancestors that gave rise to abstract thought) was present during a period of human evolution that came well before cities, agriculture, and Pokémon Go. It happened while our forebears were wandering around in small groups, foraging, hunting, and gathering.

Because our brain proved *capable* of abstract thought and complex mental abilities 50,000 to 500,000 years ago, it is by examining the selective pressures that existed then that help us understand how we developed the brains that now allow us to write novels, perform heart transplants, and fill YouTube with comments (and sometimes idiotic banter). Crabtree says it best: "Almost certainly our present day abilities are a collateral effect of being selected for more fundamental tasks."

Those tasks are almost identical to what we experience when we head outdoors into unstructured landscapes. The evidence supports the notion that from an evolutionary perspective, being outdoor hunter-gatherers required as much abstract thought as living in the present day.

As you've probably noted, I find Crabtree's research revelatory. As a teacher committed to getting kids outside, this research provides strong support for the idea that being outdoors and moving through landscapes is more than just some prehistoric footnote—it's a central component of the evolution of thinking and intelligence.

The research, if it holds up, puts the very act of outdoor education in new light. Now, obviously, over the course of *one* generation, none of this matters. But multiplied across billions of people over a couple of thousand years, and something very unprecedented could happen on a genetic level. Despite the fact that most of us now possess cheap, handheld technology that would've seemed like science fiction fifty years ago and god-like 50,000 years earlier than that—and despite the fact that we have more information at our fingertips than even our grandparents dreamed possible—we still may be regressing in terms of intelligence.

CITY LIVIN' SOFTIES

The root causes of adaptive intelligence lie in the way the stretch of our evolutionary development played out as our brains grew big. During this time—moving through open landscapes in small hunter-gatherer bands—the pressure exerted to survive was intense. We could've starved, become prey, killed each other, and simply winked out of existence like so many other species that couldn't make the cut. But we didn't. We developed intelligence because our circumstances demanded it. So what happened? Why might our intelligence now be deteriorating?

Crabtree guesses it was our agriculturally fueled, city-livin', sedentary lifestyle that did it. "When might we have begun to loss [*sic*] these abilities? Most likely we started our slide with the invention of agriculture, which enabled high density living in cities."

He also notes that our current and historical communities were mutually supportive. To some degree, as a species we all clumped together to make life a little easier. "Lapses of judgement or failure of comprehension" were less likely to get us eaten. We got soft, and so did our brains.

So what does this have to do with schools, with outdoor education? Stay with me—we're almost there.

An argument against Crabtree would be that we've got the Space Station, the iPhone, and Google's self-driving cars—all items that would had made a caveman's head spin. We're obviously smarter now, but we've been doing complex tasks for thousands of years: surviving on the savannah, building shelters in the bush, presaging seasonal changes to follow game, doing laundry, farming, playing Minecraft. These are all tasks that we accomplish just by using the big brains that we already made many years ago. "Our nervous system evolved until recently to do common, but computation complex task [*sic*] very well, hence none of our modern abilities are different than just a retrofit of modes of thought that we have been selected to do as hunter-gatherers."

Here's where the rubber hits the road. Crabtree writes: "Many kinds of modern refined intellectual activity (*that our children are judged by*) may not necessarily require more innovation, synthesis, and creativity than more ancient forms." The parentheses are his; the italics mine because I think this is a crucial bit.

We ask our children to demonstrate competency in tasks that are ill-suited to their very genetic build. This isn't to say that we haven't created intellectual marvels in the past few thousand years, nor is it to say that we should all just take kids into the woods every day and have them build atlatls and bows and hunt squirrels (though I've heard worse ideas—ahem, Common Core, I'm lookin' at you). But by understanding that our abilities as *thinkers*—as emotionally complex, intelligent beings—were wrought through an intimate relationship with our environment as hunter-gatherers, we can begin to push for a more diverse and deeper outdoor experience for our students. It's not *just* playtime out there in the woods, nor is it *only* a bit of exercise. It's a fundamental experience to our genetic frameworks, and to head outdoors with a group of kids is to step back in time to the very dawn of our imagination.

We were at the Lincoln Park Zoo in Chicago two years ago. In the big cat hall, we spotted an agitated leopard. It paced back and forth, staring with those piercing, elemental eyes toward the lion enclosure across the way. There was, oddly, no lion in sight, but still the leopard stalked back and forth, intermittently letting loose its harsh, eerie, guttural bark.

People laughed and looked startled, eyes wide with excitement to see the leopard all riled up. Phones by the dozen soaked the moment up to be posted and tweeted and shared. As I watched, I couldn't help but be struck by the incongruity of it all. That leopard was not meant to be in a small, enclosed cage with fake rocks and trees surrounded by native Chicagoans and tourists.

Leopards are the most widespread of the big cats, aren't fussy eaters, and have maintained a global presence as a species, even though we big, dumb humans have done our darndest to hunt and develop them out of existence.

Don't get me wrong—I'm a fan of zoos and understand the important role they play in education and conservation. But in that moment, I believe I understood that leopard. It wanted open landscape—to hunt, to find mates, raise young, run away. I keep remembering that moment whenever I walk by the windows of my son's school and see kids indoors, tapping away at iPads. It just doesn't fit with our evolutionary history. The leopard didn't belong there trapped behind the glass; the kids don't either.

We now reward proficiency with data management, the use of digital tools, and obsequious obedience and conscientiousness rather than the kind of abstract thinking native to our brains. Intelligences that would've prospered in our evolutionary history are now a source of distraction. What was once the very stuff of living life has been relegated to a few minutes of playtime or recess—if the kids are lucky.

Crabtree's work reminds us of what we already knew; the outdoors pushes us to be our best, most emotionally capable and intelligent selves (despite the fact that it's rooted in what is currently a rather trendy ideology—paleo— notwithstanding).

PALEOEDUCATION PEDAGOGY

The current craze for everything paleo (paleo cooking, exercising, lifestyles, and diets) has the potential to be a deeply flawed approach to understanding human behavior. The way we live now, or the ways in which we can lead better, healthier lives, is not reducible to an examination of the supposed lifestyles evident in prehistoric human culture. But it's understandable, the way we exult the hunter-gatherer lifestyle: in looking back on a pre-material, pre-institutionalized culture, we see something of our better selves (or at least we imagine we do) and seek to regain that state. This, in a nutshell, is the state of being outside, free in the open air.

In that spirit, "paleoeducation" is the direct and unstructured experience of natural environments with no intermediary influences. It's free, always available, and produces no greenhouse gases! I use the term "paleo" here somewhat playfully, knowing full well that the whole of paleo culture has a bit of commercial silliness to it, but also with the aim of aligning paleoeduca- tion with an understanding of how evolutionary biology plays a role in how we learn. I know this from personal experience.

Finn has been into archaic humans for years. I suppose it's the collateral damage of having evolution-obsessed parents and siblings. His mom studied primatology as an undergrad and his sister studied anthropology, worked in conservation biology, and now is in graduate school researching Pacific squid. Instead of watching *The Avengers* together on the weekend, we make popcorn, dim the lights, and watch BBC's "Walking with Cavemen" and the PBS series "First Peoples." We're dorks.

There is one scene in particular from the BBC series that caught Finn's interest. It's a scene of *Homo heidelbergensis* hunting an Irish elk with spears. We'd been making rock-tipped spears for years—finding spear-shaped stones and tying (and sometimes duct-taping) them into the split ends of body-length maple sapling shafts. But the scene showed *heidelbergensis* using wooden points. Finn was fascinated. He wanted to make one, and it sounded better than vacuuming out the car and folding laundry to me.

We researched how to fire-harden an ash spear point. We consulted with our octogenarian neighbor who spent his career in forestry. Ash trees, we'd read, made the best spears since they are dense, springy, and able to hold a point. Our neighbor helped us locate an ash sapling, which we cut down. We built a fire in the backyard of our condo and shaped and sharpened a length of ash with a hatchet and sandpaper. Finn patiently spent the requisite time slowly fire-hardening the point by waving it near the flames. Soon, we had a convincingly real looking, sharp, and frankly, deadly spear. We used his old archery target, and, with a running start, Finn hurled the spear at the target. It pierced the tough nylon weave of the cover and embedded itself deep in the dense padding. The tip stayed sharp, honed by the carbon of the fire.

What struck me about the experience—other than the fact that our neighbors now thought we were weirder than ever—is that Finn had so much fun without recourse to stuff made by machines. All that we needed, really, was a hatchet, and any blade would've worked.

It was so low-tech. We didn't have to buy anything. We didn't have to get in the car and drive to some place like Toys 'R Us, to be drowned by an overwhelming commercial stimuli tsunami. We had reached a moment where, if only briefly, industrially produced material things didn't matter as much. Even our other outdoor experiences—hiking, camping, boating—all require backpacks, hiking shoes, weather-resistant clothes, and cars to get us around. Rarely did we have the chance to make something, *do something*, which was so fun and didn't really require anything other than ourselves. We repeated the experiment by using another part of the sapling to shape a spear, and this time we used a sharp-edged rock to hack a point. Just to see if we could.

It was in direct contrast to many of the messages received from the larger sphere of "outdoor culture." Looking around at the outdoor lifestyle espoused by *Outside* magazine and the glossy brochures of Patagonia, prAna, and North Face, the message quickly becomes apparent: to be outdoorsy you must buy things, and in order to have the right kind of outdoor experiences, you have to spend a bunch of money on clothes, equipment, and travel. You're not a true "outdoorsman" or "outdoorswoman" unless you're clomping up a track in the Alps in fancy hiking boots, or fording a frothy current wearing wicking underlayers in Iceland, or taking in the breathtaking vistas of New Zealand clad in sustainable wool pantaloons.

This consumer-driven philosophy can trickle down to our students. In fact, the message is so pervasive in our culture that we think that taking children out to climb the trees that fringe a nearby vacant lot is somehow a cheapened version of real adventure. The locations and gear need to have some cachet, apparently, to have educational validity. This is where paleoeducation comes into play by acting against this commercial narrative; reducing the required materials down to that which can be found, not bought, and replacing travel to exotic places with the exploration of our own backyards. In fact, repeated experiences in the unstructured, natural world can accrue within a student's worldview and lead to a redesignation of priorities—if one is willing to subject them to a bit of backcountry rambling.

In my experience as a teacher, helping students navigate this shift—seeing education as a process of experience rather than one of consumption—was brought to light most clearly on one particular backpacking trip in the High Sierra.

To be fair, it *had* been a particularly exhausting trip. Leaving the lodge's parking lot a week before, the dozen or so middle schoolers and I had humped up snow-choked passes and vertiginous switch-backed trails. We'd eaten every last molecule of sugar we possessed. We were grimy, tired, and spent. By the time we limped back into the campsite, we had reached that odd state that comes after a decent patch spent in the wilderness. We were tired, sure, but also stronger. The packs on our backs—though lighter than they'd been when we began—no longer felt all that heavy. Walking up trails at altitudes above 8,000 feet no longer made black spots pop before our eyes, and our breath didn't ratchet up into gasping low gear as it had before. We were sapped to our baseline, but our baseline was in many ways arguably stronger and fitter than it had been the week previous.

It felt good. And it felt even better that our ride was coming the next day to take us home. Darkness settled in, and everyone gratefully began to yawn and stretch and get ready for bed.

Some students just flopped down in their sleeping bags on the ground while others used foam mats. Another slept on top of the picnic table. No one pitched tents. I hoped it wouldn't rain.

I didn't think much of it at the time since it wasn't long before I myself succumbed to sleep. But I think back to that trip and those specific moments before we all fell asleep every once and awhile. What occurs to me is that often the argument we make about outdoor education—especially the rigorous, extended adventure sort—is that it makes students *appreciate* their worldly comforts more. That by enforcing a synthetic bare-bones existence in the wild, kids will be more grateful for their material abundance. They'll be more appreciative of the wonders of the industrialized world, and stop taking everything for granted.

But that's wrong, actually. Our goal should be to *depreciate* the value of material culture.

"I'll bet you'll be glad to get home, eat food on the couch, and watch your shows!" parents would say upon picking up their stinky, bug-bitten kids from these trips. And, of course, the kids would be looking forward to those diversions. But really, what the outdoors can do—*should* do—is get kids to see that really, those things are unnecessary. It's a stark example, but the comfort we think we derive from beds and sleeping indoors and always having food available and never having to carry anything ourselves is a false comfort. What the students got a taste of during that moment when they heaped themselves around the campsite was the reality that much of their material world was unnecessary. For a moment, the value of their material world was not intrinsic, but a fabrication of consent.

We *need* this new toaster because it toasts faster. We *need* a second car because our schedules are so hectic and we live so far away from work. We *need* to experience the outdoors through expensive sports like alpine skiing, dependent on technology, fossil fuels, and a ton of gear. This line of thinking can bring education to its knees as new technologies are seen as requirements to the learning process. Students as well begin to view learning as the dividend of accessing more complicated and powerful technological tools, rather than accessing the limitlessness of their own imagination and experience. And in addition, this equation is exactly what has gotten us into the environmental mess we're in—and the way to get out of it is to drop everything and head back outside.

SAYING FAREWELL TO THE VAQUITA

The fact is that being outdoors leads to an awareness of the inherent nature of other species and their value. We realize that we are not apart from nature, but intertwined with it. It is not Man versus Wild—it is Man *and* Wild (excuse the gender bias). No matter how much we educate children about conservation, recycling, climate change, or pollution, we still rely on the same systems, institutions, and tools that caused the degradation of natural environments so that they need conserving. We try as educators, parents, and human beings who give a rat's ass about the future to try and solve these problems using the same technologies and cultural structures that produced the problems in the first place.

The only way to teach kids real environmental awareness is through a radical rejection of the very tools that screwed everything up in the first place.

Being outdoors—radically free of the indoor world and its demands—leads to a depreciation of the imagined necessity of material culture.

In reality, the situation is rather grim. There are simply too many people on the planet, consuming too many resources. It's untenable. The only solution is within the next generation of Americans—our kids, our students—and their revolutionary rejection of material culture. In this way, the fate of the world rests with teachers. But what can they do? What can parents do?

It's likely that during their lifetime my children, Finn and Vivien, will say goodbye to the Amur Tiger, the world's largest cat. What part of our imagination will die with it? Sumatran elephant, western lowland gorilla, vaquita (the world's most endangered sea mammal) are all likely to disappear from the face of the planet in the next few years. How do we solve this brutally destabilizing disconnect? What can teachers and parents do? How do we insert a *paleo* ethos into education?

I have a few ideas:

Go Outside with Your Kids All the Time

This seems simple, but it's not. When I taught middle school students in a dense suburb of Los Angeles, I was reprimanded for bringing my students outside too much. In typical nose-thumbing fashion, I responded by instituting physical education for almost ninety junior high students every morning. We'd walk through city streets to nearby parks where kids could climb trees, play soccer, or just sit in the grass. It was a rather dicey proposition. Once, a student got in a fistfight with a pedestrian who had made some unsavory comments about her hair—but we persevered. It can be done.

Smash Your Screens

This will no doubt send you into apoplectic shivers. *No, not my precious iPhone!* Adults claim they need their phones for work. Schools especially invest billions of dollars in educational technology, usually in the form of computers. However, according to a recent report from the Organisation for Economic Co-operation and Development (the OECD is an international research consortium with over thirty participating countries), computers don't necessarily improve student learning: "Despite considerable investments in computers, Internet connections and software for educational use, there is little solid evidence that greater computer use among students leads to better scores in mathematics and reading."

Of the many demands we've made of teachers and schools over the past few decades, getting our children indoctrinated with the latest enviro-consciousness has been one of the most prevalent. While we expect schools to be able to do it, going outside with your kids and getting away from screens is markedly more successful than getting schools to imbue your child with some sense of environmental awareness. Despite how we may hope that school will "teach" our children about nature, it's a hit or miss proposition. Some do, and do it well—with spirit and compassion and vision. Some don't or do it poorly. The reality is that direct exposure to nature—moments of direct contact—can be the most powerful learning moments a child can have.

Change the Outdoor Education Approach

Many environmental educators have done the best job they can to introduce kids of all kinds to nature and the outdoor world. Everyone I've ever met that works at nature centers or as an environmental educator is earnest, well-meaning, kind, and committed to a general environmental stewardship and consciousness that I can totally get behind. But to deny that environmental education as it stands isn't in need of some shifts is wrong.

Until a few decades ago, there wasn't even such a concept as "environmental education." Back in the mid-twentieth century, Americans were still glee-fully chopping and mining and polluting the heck out of the natural world. In 1969, there was the infamous Cuyahoga River fire in Cleveland, when an oil spill on the water actually ignited, causing over $100,000 in damage. It was, ironically, at a time when cleanup of the Cuyahoga was a priority for the powers that be in Cleveland. While that particular fire made the city and river one of the epicenters of the nascent environmental movement, the river had been catching fire for decades.

As environmental education became part of curriculums in both elementary and secondary school and colleges, the question of how to teach kids—particularly those in urban and suburban neighborhoods—became a central question within the environmental movement. Or, rather, it *should* have become a central question, but instead most environmental educators (including yours truly, when I taught middle school science in the early 2000s) borrowed their approach and theory and philosophy from the conservation movement.

Ever since John Muir segregated the "wildness" of places like Yosemite in 1890, the conservation movement as well as large-scale environmental ethos of the United States has been impractical. The notion that large swaths of wilderness—parks, wildlife refuges, forests, deserts, and mountains—need to be returned to some idyllic "pristine" state is a myth. As any anthropologist will point out, people have been living within just about every ecosystem on our continent for thousands of years, from the frigid northern reaches of the polar ice cap to the sweltering tropics and everything in between. The idea that we need to return nature to some primeval, peopleless state is false and misleading. It also sets us up for a radical separation from the very thing we want to save.

The environmental education movement has echoed these unattainable goals, raising nature and "wilderness" up on a pedestal that removes it from the daily experience of children.

In an essay from the book *Children & Nature*, David Sobel—whose research has focused on children's unstructured play in the natural world—says of the urge kids have to climb trees, explore bird's nests, walk across beaver dams, and pull apart milkweed pods in their never-ending exploration for novelty in the natural world:

> This is the joy of children encountering the natural world on their own terms, and more and more it is becoming a lost idyll, no longer an integral part of growing up. There are many reasons for this loss—urbanization, the changing social structure of families, tick-and mosquito-borne illness, the fear of stranger-danger. And perhaps even environmental education is one of the cause of children's alienation from nature.

It's counterintuitive to be sure—this thought that the very organizations, teachers, and policies bent on getting children to engage with nature in the hopes that they become stewards of the natural landscape are actually degrading kids' ability to connect in an authentic, important way with nature. And yet we see this all the time—in the way nature is described as this pristine, untouchable phenomenon; distant and categorized, fragile and valuable. It's rather like the baubles and ceramic figurines your old aunt would keep on a shelf that your parents warned you *not to touch*.

Sobel writes: "Much of environmental education today has taken on a museum mentality, where nature is a composed exhibit on the other side of the glass." This is true to a large extent, and my own experience as an educator supports his claim. I remember working at an urban school in Pasadena, California. Two incidents stand out in my mind.

Once I took my students on a hike up a nearby canyon. Hardly pristine wilderness, the canyon was a mere sixteen miles from downtown LA. During this hike, kids ran and screamed, or sullenly kicked up dust as they unwillingly marched along to the waterfall at the end of the hike. But some played in the trickling river that ran down out of the San Gabriel Mountains. Others actually got completely soaked in the falls themselves, standing under the pouring water surrounded by the screams and encouragement of other students.

In one particular section of trail, the buzz of a disturbed rattlesnake could be heard from a rocky crevice, and the students that heard it shied away, eyes wide with fear and sparkling with a kind of rejuvenation that wasn't normally available in our small classroom back at school. A few kids got stabbed by the sharp spines of yucca plants. Others got a bit parched because they'd ignored advice to bring water. It was real, and, though it only lasted an afternoon, I wondered what the result would be of prolonged, intimate contact with a landscape like this. If I had the time in my teaching to really engage them in this landscape, what would they think of it?

The second experience was not as much fun. Or, more accurately, not fun at all. Someone who had held my position previously had ordered these "earth science kits"—boxes of group activities that simulated ecosystems and geology. I dug them out of a huge container that lurked, heavy and metal and gray, in the corner of the school parking lot. I brought them to class and set up the activities for groups of students. It was what I refer to as "chaos" education, a phrase borrowed from film reviewers to describe animated feature films that are all noise and funny voices and explosions and constant stimuli to engage the jittery minds of overstimulated kids.

The class was filled with vinegar and baking soda volcanos and various experiments. I practically tore my hair out trying to get them to do the experiments "correctly," and by the end of the day my class was a mess, I was exhausted, and the students may not have learned a damn thing.

Much of the problem was probably mine. I was in my mid-twenties at the time and didn't have the experience to orchestrate a lesson with those little kits to a room of forty kids in a way that made sense. But on the other hand, when I took them on that little ramble up the canyon, it was so *easy*. I felt guilty, like I was taking the day off. But students from that time, which was almost fifteen years ago now, still remember the angry, hornet-like buzz of the rattler. The way Mark Lopez was the first to leap into the pounding waterfall and get soaked. How yucca has quite the effective defense system. The way sun and exertion make you thirsty.

In one of his autobiographical reminiscences, biologist E. O. Wilson wrote:

> Hands-on experience at the critical time, not systematic knowledge, is what counts in the making of a naturalist. Better to be an untutored savage for a while, not to know the names or anatomical detail. Better to spend long stretches of time just searching and dreaming.

Paleoeducation is a step in exactly this direction. By reducing the engagement students have with the natural world to a very direct, dirty, and curiosity-driven method, we form the foundation for understanding, rather than imposing the arbitrary rules of abstract, scientific reasoning. When students splash through a stream, flipping over rocks, they come to an innate understanding of the physics of liquids; they investigate weird little invertebrates clinging to the underside of river stones; they absorb the interplay between water, earth, sun, and plants. There is so much happening all around them, and they can soak it up at their own pace, in their own way, and build on that tacit understanding later, when larger, theory-driven ideas like ecosystems and the water cycle are taught because in essence they *know* about them already. Terminology and theory are easy if students are given firsthand experience to bolster the acquisition of knowledge.

Paleoeducational models are particularly adept at this. Being outdoors allows kids to engage in the style and type of learning they are designed for; exploratory, unstructured, fun, and collaborative. Paleoeducation is simply immersing the students in the natural world and allowing the terrain, their investigations, the course of the sun through the sky, the weather, and their own bodies' natural limitations to guide their learning.

Chapter 3

Feral Psychology

Nomad Youth is a camp where kids explore the rivers, lakes, and mountains of Vermont. It's fun, of course, but also instructive. The structure of the camp—if it can be called structure—is to head out each morning to some wild spot and then play for a few hours, eat lunch, wander around, collect sticks and rocks, and then eventually head home.

It's worth mentioning that I created Nomad Youth for my son and his friends. Normally, I would find the idea of providing child care and supervision to a car load of yelling elementary schoolchildren a rather daunting task. But I wanted my son, Finn, to have the sort of experiences I remembered as a kid; long rambles in the woods, playing in rivers, and exploring the world around me with minimal interference from adults. Car rides with tween-pop blasting my eardrums seemed a small price to pay for providing Finn and his friends with these sorts of outdoor excursions.

Research strongly suggests that being outdoors—in non-developed, natural environments—has a positive effect on the behavior of children. A National Wildlife Federation report states that outdoor play helps kids lead healthier lives and reduces stress, lessens anxiety, and generates a greater sense of personal freedom. The report concludes that outdoor time can lead to happier kids—something parents intuitively know from experience. An article from the *Sydney Morning Herald* quotes a pediatrician in an article about how outdoor time makes for more stable young people:

> Dr. Kathleen Berchelmann sees the most extreme cases of stressed, depressed and anxious kids. At least once a week, she says, she cares for a teenager who has tried to commit suicide.
>
> "It's frightening," said Berchelmann, a pediatric specialist at Barnes-Jewish, Missouri Baptist and Progress West hospitals. When she inquires about healthy

activities in the teens' lives, almost none mention anything outdoors. They went to summer camp once, they say, and that was wonderful.

Berchelmann said she notices her most carefree patients have opposite lives. They are covered in ticks after being out catching frogs, got a hook stuck in their ear while fishing in a creek or have an infected mosquito bite after a camping trip.

"They are the ones waiting an hour to see you and are still giggling when you get in the room," she said.

We know that being outside is good for our bodies (including our brains)—but what about our minds? Or, if we want to delve into the occult, what about that ethereal thing known as "the spirit"?

Both in reviewing the research and exploring our own anecdotal experience, it seems clear that nature leads to feelings of well-being. But could it be that our default setting is actually one of happy, optimistic contentment?

Maybe it's not the *outdoors* making us well; maybe it's the *indoors* making us sick.

THE OUTDOOR PRESCRIPTION

The question in psychology should be what is the relationship between being locked inside all day and the leading psychological illnesses? The link between spending time outdoors and alleviating depression seems clear. One wonders about anxiety, obsessive compulsive disorder, schizotypal disorders, narcissism, and other personality disorders. How many are caused by the oppressive structure of the indoors and all its concurrent restraint? While many of those psychological conditions have multiple causes, including genetic disorders, it seems possible, indeed probable, that too much time indoors can adversely affect our overall temperament and psychological balance.

And what about children? According to the National Center for Learning Disabilities (NCLD), one-third of children who suffer from various learning disabilities such as dyslexia or visual processing deficit also have ADHD. The NCLD notes that ADHD can be treated with various "behavioral" and "pharmacological" therapies. No doubt many children who toil under the onus of ADHD benefit from drug therapy. It also seems likely that there is a hereditary component to ADHD, as well as links to brain structure and neurochemical imbalances. However, it is also true that simply getting students who have ADHD outside more often has improved their performance and ameliorated the symptoms of ADHD. And not just ADHD improves with time outdoors; the treatment of depression, anxiety, and other behaviors and conditions has positive results with the application of time outdoors.

Conventionally, we've separated pursuits of the body—sports, exercise, and health—with the abilities of the brain—cognition, memory, and analysis. This division (the old mind–body conundrum) has been thoroughly debunked through research. In fact, movement is so closely associated with learning and thinking that the two are often used to describe each other. In *Mind Change*, a book about how our screen-based culture may be changing our brains, neuroscientist Susan Greenfield writes:

> The crucial issue here is how we digest internally what is happening around us as we travel through each day. The Austrian physician who developed the current treatment for Parkinson's disease back in the 1960's, Oleh Hornykiewicz, once offered this insight: "Thinking is movement confined to the brain." A movement is characterized by a chain of linked actions that take place in a particular order. The simplest example, walking, is a series of steps in which placing one foot forward leads to the other foot overtaking it. One step leads to the next in a cause-and-effect chain that is not random but a fixed linear sequence. So it is with thought.

OUTDOOR CHIVALRY

Perhaps one way to look at the way the outdoors can engender a positive frame of mind—even one in which behavior is modified to include more compassionate and empathetic attributes—is to look at an example of *yearning to do good*. Some of the best examples can be found in various *bildungsroman* novels.

Middlemarch is widely held to be George Eliot's (the pen name of Mary Ann Evans) masterpiece. It's a pretty solid conjecture. I don't know of many other novels that capture the vicissitudes of life, abject failure, prideful ignorance, and our own ability to deceive ourselves and suffer the consequences as brilliantly as in *Middlemarch*. The book's engaging, varied cast members are a riotously fascinating assemblage, and the vast scope of the book creates a world of its own within the page-bound environs of *Middlemarch*.

Not so *Daniel Deronda*, Eliot's last book, her most ambitious, and, if you ask me, ultimate triumph as a writer. The two main characters—the eponymous Daniel Deronda and the maddeningly capricious Gwendolyn Grandcourt—seem to me to be two of the most finely drawn portraits of real human beings I've ever read in a novel. *Middlemarch* may have captured the random and vulgar change that wreaks havoc on us all, but *Daniel Deronda* dives deep into our souls and demonstrates how infinite our capacities for self-reflection really are.

Deronda is a man of the landed gentry—sort of. His benefactor, the nobleman Sir Hugo, acts as a kind and compassionate uncle. Deronda doesn't know who his parents were, and suspects that part of the reason is that it's in fact Sir Hugo that is secretly his father, with Deronda as the illegitimate son. The mystery of Deronda's origins plagues him. He is too overwhelmed with fear of the truth to ask Sir Hugo himself—but Sir Hugo is fond of him and treats him well, raising him, in most respects, as one would a son.

But as he's not Sir Hugo's son (as far as we know as we read the book) Deronda will not inherit title or land. He must make his own way in the world. As an unofficial nobleman, Deronda is acutely aware of his uselessness. The banality of social obligation as Sir Hugo's favorite weighs heavily upon him, and he goes from drawing room to balls to "town," feeling the stultifying oppression of being an upstanding member of the aristocracy without much purpose.

But Deronda seeks meaning in his life as ferociously as any character in literature. He finds it by befriending a strange, semi-hermit Jew who spouts mystical pronouncements and by saving the life of a poor woman who tries to drown herself. Deronda is truly a knight errant, looking desperately for purpose, intensely eager to enact his goodness upon the world.

Deronda is the perfect symbol for the shackles we've put on children by keeping them indoors. The outdoors—hiking, swimming, or just crashing around the woods—brings about countless opportunities for chivalry. Believe me, I'm as skeptical of waxing romantic as Sancho Panza, but the reality is that for us to create good citizens, we have to provide opportunities for independent acts of sacrifice and goodness. Sometimes it comes down to sharing your last Oreo with a friend on a long hike; sometimes it's taking some weight from the pack of a suffering fellow hiker. Situations where we're offered the chance to come to the aid of someone else abound in unstructured, outdoor environments. Cold? Borrow my jacket. Tired? I'll carry your pack for a bit. Blistered? Let me dig out my bandages and patch you up.

R-E-S-P-E-C-T!

One of the words you hear a lot in education that I've been trying to wrap my head around is "respect." All over my kid's school there are posters driving home the concept of respect. "Respect ourselves, respect each other, respect our school," reads one such poster. Once, when I was picking my son up from second grade and the hallways were packed with a mad scrum of elementary students, banging every which way with overloaded SpongeBob Squarepants backpacks, I heard a teacher yell, "Respectful bodies, please!" with vehemence. The kids dutifully slowed as though they understood, but I was confused. The ultimate respect we can show our bodies is to move them about, often and with abandon.

I've had to break up far fewer confrontations outdoors than in the classroom. When I taught elementary and middle school, I will admit that I was not a very good classroom "manager" (and what a terrible term). I replaced mediation and compromise with volume and repetition, as in "Sit down, Steven. Now. Sit! Sit. Down. Now!" I've seen teachers much, much better than I create a calming classroom culture. But I've also seen how tired they are, how exhausted. Kids, stuck inside, with a bunch of *things* to argue over (my eraser! my book! my turn on the computer!) will indeed argue. But outdoors there's less to argue about—there's more space and less things of imagined value. You want to play with a stick? Go ahead. There's plenty to go around.

But it's more than that, and while I may be accused of being starry-eyed, I think it bears on our discussion. There's a chance to do good—real, actual, good—in unstructured natural environments. Kids help each other to scramble over logs, build forts together, and hold hands crossing the slippery rocks in a river. They provide camaraderie, share stories, and laugh *together*, not at each other.

When we put them indoors, they're like Daniel Deronda, desperate for meaning, for purpose, for the chance to truly be heroes. We all want to be heroic, at some level. Being inside the classroom is just like the suffocating atmosphere of the Victorian drawing room: all arbitrary rules and etiquette and boring decorum. What kids want is the chance to be great, to let their best selves shine. Like Deronda, they are trapped by obligation. By forcing kids to constantly be indoors, we run the risk of turning them into someone like Henleigh Grandcourt, Deronda's snobbish nemesis who finds just about everything a "frightful bore."

In *Philosophical Issues in Adventure Education* by Scott Wurdinger, the author details this very notion—that an outdoor environment, given its inherent challenges and natural venues for teamwork, can actually spur just the kind of altruism and good work demonstrated by characters like Deronda. Wurdinger writes: "One must be exposed to risk-taking situations in order to learn to act courageously." Given the competitive nature of our classrooms, it is challenging in a traditional, indoors environment to create these avenues for bravery.

"Participants are faced with challenges which require action, and these acts are often compassionate, courageous, and just," Wurdinger writes. Furthermore, what becomes clear is that while in the classroom it is the content, or method of instruction, that takes the center stage. In the outdoors the very personality and character of the teacher takes on a higher importance. We begin to teach by being, rather than telling—the most powerful tool there is in terms of teaching by relationship. Just as Deronda instructs through fictionalized example, so too does the outdoor teacher have myriad opportunities to demonstrate selflessness, courage, and kindness. "This implies," writes

Wurdinger, "that the teacher's personality, which is not a part of the formal curriculum, has tremendous potential to affect moral development."

Research seems to strongly support the idea that being outdoors, in natural environments, not only provides real context-dependent situations for demonstrating altruism, generosity, and kindness, but that the change that occurs when individuals are outdoors is even deeper on a psychological level. Researchers from the University of Rochester published a study that is indicative of the types of psychological shifts we're talking about—a kind of natural history of Deronda-ization that can take place when we surround ourselves with nature. The article, "Can Nature Make Us More Caring? Effects of Immersion in Nature on Intrinsic Aspirations and Generosity," specifically addresses the way that being in natural, outdoor environments shifts our focus from *extrinsic* to *intrinsic* aspirations. Extrinsic aspirations are exactly what they sound like: stuff we aspire to that exists outside of ourselves, like a sweet Rolex watch, fawning groupies, killer abs, bling, Benz—you get the idea. Conversely, intrinsic aspirations are the stuff of personal development: personal growth, fostering real relationships, and trying to be a better person.

A key point in the study is that folks who are immersed in nature value personal growth over things primarily because of an increased feeling of "personal autonomy." The researchers define it thus: "Autonomy is experienced as being in touch with oneself or having a sense of inner congruence and self-authorship, and freedom from external and internal pressures."

In higher education, we often ask students to reflect upon what they *think*—no doubt a valuable exercise, and arguably the basis for all critical introspection and analysis. This sort of self-reflection is key in figuring out personal ethics and beliefs. However, we don't often have the opportunity to ask students to reflect on what they've *done*, or what *happened*. Or, more succinctly, we don't get the chance to have them reflect on *experiences* as much.

Yes, learning things in a classroom, watching films, attending lectures, and having discussions are all experiences. But they are usually classically didactic; we watch the movie *Rabbit Proof Fence* as a means of understanding the way education has been used as a tool in colonial imperialism to disenfranchise indigenous Australian aborigines, for example. Experience in the outdoors has a tendency to be messy, non-linear, and harder to grapple with. And, I'd argue, more valuable in some ways as a platform for just this kind of self-reflection that leads to a greater valuation of intrinsic aspirations.

The researchers remind us that autonomy is derived from these types of outdoor experiences because they offer unique "opportunities to integrate experience by encouraging introspection and a coherent sense of self" in part because in the woodsy or unpeopled stretches of the world, we can get away from the buzz of institutional responsibility and remind ourselves that it actually matters who we are.

THE CRANKY SQUATTER

Thanks to a keen local interest in maintaining a steady stream of incoming tourists, it's not hard to envision what mid-nineteenth-century Concord Massachusetts looked like during the time that Ralph Waldo Emerson, Louisa May Alcott, and Henry David Thoreau called it their home. Many of the original buildings from that period still stand and have kept up 1800s appearances. A number of years ago my family and I visited the town and took a tour of Emerson's house, now a museum. Finn, then about three, crawled under the velvet guard ropes in one of the rooms while the tour guide gave a dusty lecture on the domestic life of the Emersons. Finn crawled under a table and fell asleep there. I'm not sure if Emerson would've been charmed, but I think his longtime tenant and friend, Thoreau, would have been.

Thoreau, author of such lodestone American standards as *Walden* and *Civil Disobedience*, was playful with children but crankily cagey with adults; brilliant yet hesitant about entering into the full intellectual stream of the day, preferring to wander the fields and woods near Concord. His writing would go on to shape not just the Transcendentalist movement but also American Romanticism and thought for the next 150 years.

The original hippie, Thoreau was anti-establishment, anti-slavery, a feminist (he welcomed the Concord Female Anti-Slavery society to his little cabin in the woods during his time at Walden pond), and a truculent citizen, but devoted friend and brother. Even Emerson, his mentor and closest friend, found him confusing.

Thoreau was certainly not an easy person to get along with. Even in literary hindsight he comes across as somewhat of an extremist. A radical individualist who was pretty cranky about, well, just about everything: government, company, farming, history, travel—even eating nice meals was anathema to the strange, ascetic version of living in nature that Thoreau represents in *Walden*. In a masterfully written takedown of him in *The New Yorker*, journalist Kathryn Schultz writes, "Why, given Thoreau's hypocrisy, his sanctimony, his dour asceticism, and his scorn, do we continue to cherish *Walden*?" It's a fair question. But rather than focus on Thoreau's literary merits, or whether or not he deserves his throne in the pantheon of American nature writing, it's helpful for us to use his life as a way to explore how nature can heal—and what that could mean for outdoor education.

WOODSY MEDICINE

Thoreau was born in 1817. One of the major events in his life came about when he was twenty-five. His brother, John, contracted tetanus from a cut on his finger he got while shaving, and died after an agonizing battle with the disease in 1842. Three years later, Thoreau would decamp from the gossipy, upwardly mobile streets of Concord and relocate to his tiny cabin near Walden Pond, which he built on land owned by Emerson.

Literary psychoanalysis is an enterprise fraught with danger. We don't know, nor really can we ever know, the true state of Thoreau's mind after his brother died. However, he left a massive pile of journals, loads of correspondence to family and friends, and his essays and books as a legacy. Through these, it is possible to tease out some possibilities about Thoreau's state of mind after losing his brother, whom he dearly loved.

In a 2014 review of *The Adventures of Henry David*, a biography written by Michael Sims, *Washington Post* reviewer Scott Russell Sanders writes that after his brother John's death, Thoreau was plunged into a "profound depression." Losing his brother upended Thoreau in a way that potentially caused him pitch in any attempt at living within society and retreat to the balm of the woods (even if said balm was only a few miles outside of town near a railway).

Thoreau wrote about his moods often, and it seems likely that—if not formally diagnosed as depressed—he certainly shares many symptoms with what we'd now label "clinical depression." In an intriguing study titled *Thoreau's Democratic Withdrawal*, by Shannon L. Mariotti, the author wrestles with the notion of Thoreau's discontent through an analysis of his iconic essay, "Walking." Responding to a passage of the essay in which Thoreau, who is sullenly marching along, ruminates on his jealous feelings toward a rooster who greets the day with a joyful and trumpeting crow, Mariotti writes:

> Compared to the rooster, who is well, Thoreau is unwell. Depressed, he likens himself to a "watcher in the house of mourning," rather than experiencing the awakening that makes it morning no matter what the clock says.

We know through Thoreau's writing that he was cranky about the modernization of society—it was one of his major themes. He felt that humans had lost some level of dignity, self-reliance, and compassionate relation to nature and each other through the fanatical industry that defined New England in the mid-1800s. Later in the analysis, Mariotti sums up Thoreau's darkly obstreperous point of view in "Walking" thus:

> First, clearly Thoreau is in town, in the village, when he hears the cock crow, for he is on a wooden sidewalk. He is downtown, most likely on a main street in Concord. He is at the epicenter of the very place where the changes wrought by modernization are the most evident.

Thoreau's thoughts darken even more. He wonders how shopkeepers, who sit about all day with "crossed legs," can bear their lives without committing suicide. And while we can't know for sure how much of Thoreau's writing was crafted with the deliberate effect of making us see our narrator as dark and edgily morbid, we can be sure that when his brother John died, Thoreau was sent into a tailspin that resulted—either consciously or subconsciously—in his leaving the noisy streets of Concord and heading into the woods.

In fact, nearly a decade after building his little cabin in the woods, when Thoreau published *Walden*, he provides us with a tidy description of what compelled him to turn his back on society and head into the woods (though we know that he was actually still a part of society, traveling back and forth to town and having guests). This is arguably one of the most famous bits of American essayistic scribbling ever, and it's quoted at length to give us ample evidence of Thoreau's depression, and subsequent transformation under a bower of pines.

> I went to the woods because I wished to live deliberately, to front only the essential facts of life, and see if I could not learn what it had to teach, and not, when I came to die, discover that I had not lived. I did not wish to live what was not life, living is so dear; nor did I wish to practice resignation, unless it was quite necessary. I wanted to live deep and suck out all the marrow of life, to live so sturdily and Spartan-like as to put to rout all that was not life, to cut a broad swath and shave close, to drive life into a corner, and reduce it to its lowest terms, and, if it proved to be mean, why then to get the whole and genuine meanness of it, and publish its meanness to the world; or if it were sublime, to know it by experience, and be able to give a true account of it in my next excursion.

Throughout this passage, Thoreau tells us why, two years after his brother's awful death, he chucks it all and decides to live in the woods by himself. "Nor did I wish to practice resignation, unless it was quite necessary." One can only imagine the feelings and circumstances that gave rise to that line. It seems entirely possible that by "resignation" what Thoreau is talking about is depression—perhaps even suicide, something that we know he thought actively about as evidenced in "Walking." His philosophical conundrum—whether or not life is "mean" or has some redeeming qualities—sounds very much like the level of desperation reached by many in the grips of depression.

Depression leads to a debate about the very point of life itself. Thoreau is grappling with this very question, whether or not life's worth living. He even, perhaps, tells us why he is in the depths of such despair, by inserting the phrase "shave close," which maybe is an unconscious nod to his brother's death. Regardless, in the utter exhaustion comprehended only by the deeply, intractably depressed person, Thoreau sees his only chance at salvation in the quiet solitude of woodsy isolation.

THE SCHOOL OF DEPRESSION

Depression is on the rise in school-age children. In fact, next to learning disorders such as ADHD, depression and its often-comorbid companion, anxiety, are reaching scary levels throughout schools. According to a survey that collected data from 2007 to 2010 by the Centers for Disease Control and Prevention, over 5 percent of boys aged twelve to seventeen suffer from depression. The number jumps to around 8 percent for girls. The result has been to medicate an entire generation of children and adults. One study in *JAMA Psychiatry*, a peer-reviewed journal published by the American Medical Association, claims that in the early 2000s antidepressant drug use jumped 36 percent per year for kids between six and seventeen years old.

It's not just better diagnostic tools or an overzealous effect to diagnose—a 2010 article from *Psychology Today* looked at longitudinal studies and found that young people were, on the whole, developing more and more cases of depression than ever before. The article states, "Today, by at least some estimates, five to eight times as many high school and college students meet the criteria for diagnosis of major depression and/or anxiety disorder as was true half a century or more ago. This increased psychopathology is not the result of changed diagnostic criteria; it holds even when the measures and criteria are constant."

At the front lines of this battle are teachers and parents, trying desperately to understand this rise in depression and the resulting decline in school performance and general well-being in our nation's youth. Saddled with federal- and state-mandated curriculum with minimal resources, teachers are also faced with a multitude of mental health issues, ranging from suicidal depression to anxiety. Teachers are educators, not mental health professionals. It's hard enough to get eleven-year-olds to understand long division, let alone help them work through complicated mental issues on the side. And yet, increasingly, that is exactly what teachers—and parents, for that matter—are faced with. The answer is usually to prescribe medication.

As a culture, facing the rising tide of depression in our nation's youth has to be a top priority. In the aforementioned *Psychology Today* article, author Peter Gray—who has written influentially about the need to remove authoritarian structure from schools—suggests that a lack of agency and self-determination may be one of the causes of depression in young people. And another possibility has emerged in recent years, causing a flurry of debate and, no doubt, some sweaty palms in the meeting rooms of GlaxoSmithKline and Merck Pharmaceuticals: maybe depression shouldn't be medicated at all; maybe it's an adapted, evolutionary trait.

Maybe it's good for us.

Depression has been noted in just about every culture, including modern hunter-gatherer cultures that live in a manner thought to be closest to our species' evolutionary origins. In order for depression to survive, the thinking goes, it must have some value to our survival as a species. Of course, this sounds counterintuitive: depression would seem to be the opposite of a survival adaptation. So what gives?

One of the researchers investigating the evolutionary roots of depression is Paul Andrews at McMaster University in Ontario, Canada. After only a few minutes on the phone with him, two things became starkly clear: Andrews is a passionate and brilliant ideologue blazing a radical path through the tangled thickets of assumptions about depression, and he's an excellent teacher. Even I, a nonexpert, was able to wrap my head around Andrews' complex theories due to his patient and methodical explanation.

The first thing that Andrews described to me is "rumination." Basically, rumination is deep, independent, solitary thought focused on a complex problem. It often is a part of depression, but as Andrews points out, it's really just a step along the trajectory we experience during a depressive episode. But, he warns, "you can't talk about rumination as a single construct," meaning that like depression itself, rumination is complex and multifaceted—there's no stand-alone definition of either phenomena.

Andrews walked me through how western medicine has come to view depression. For a long time it's been labeled as "pathological and cyclical," according to Andrews, and treated as such. It has been viewed, particularly within the last few decades, as an illness to be mitigated with either therapy or medication.

But in conducting his studies, Andrews began to see correlations between rumination—again, the deep-thinking process associated with depression—and an "analytical processing style." Rumination as a component of depression was analytical in structure, Andrews stated, because it accomplished the following steps:

1. Helps you understand the nature of your problem.
2. Helps determine why the problem occurred.
3. Generates potential solutions.
4. Evaluates potential solutions.

Numbers 1 and 2 are what Andrews refers to as the "what/problem" step, whereas numbers 3 and 4 are the "why/solution" part of the equation.

Rumination helps with complex problems in particular because the solution to the problem is not immediately apparent. For the mathematically minded out there, the equation would look something like this:

Complex Problems + Depression + Rumination = Problem Solving

Andrews argues that in general, this sequence is "self-limiting," meaning that it is a controlled loop of sorts, and potentially even cyclical. It's possible that there are problems that are so complex that no amount of rumination can solve them, but for most cases of depression something like the aforementioned steps appear to be intrinsic.

The difficulty in making Andrews' view jibe with typical conceptions about depression is that the way we think about depression isn't entirely accurate. We depend on generally held notions and popular opinions about depression, rather than really analyzing what goes on during a bout with depression for most people. Andrews noted that we have a "veneer of truth" about depression that we all understand, but it doesn't fit with the research.

For instance, the first doubts I had about depression being an evolutionary adaptation came in the form of appetite. One of the reasons we may get kind of cranky when we're hungry is that crankiness—or aggressiveness—is an evolutionary advantage when food is scarce. Just think of your kids, howling and snarling in the backseat when you pass by the exit with Subway and Chipotle, tears of resentment pouring down their face and you'll agree: hunger leads to some very forceful, effective behaviors. But people that are depressed don't eat, right? Wrong. Well, sort of wrong.

According to Andrews, "They do eat, they just eat less." He also brought up a connected but equally interesting point about how depressed people eat; they pound more carbohydrates. Think about it. If you've ever suffered a depressive episode—and according to the Anxiety and Depression Association of America, some 18 million adults suffer from depression, which when added to other anxiety disorders cost the nation a whopping $42 billion each year—then you know that when depressed, we eat carbs.

While not necessarily clinically depressed, I, like lots of folks, have experienced intense depression. And when it happened, I ate pizza, pasta, french fries—comfort foods that happened to be loaded with carbs. This is smart from an evolutionary point of view. If depression allows us to work through complex problems, best to eat those foods that provide the most direct source of long-burning fuel. Just like athletes who "carbo-load" before an endurance event, depressed people have evolved to eat more carbohydrates when depressed.

The other seemingly incongruous issue is sleep. Depressed people have irregular sleep patterns, oftentimes hardly sleeping at all. But they do sleep; they only sleep less, according to the research. The idea of the classic melancholic, sleeplessly wasting away their lives, is not entirely accurate. Yes, their food consumption habits change, and yes, their sleep patterns change. But in general, they eat and sleep enough to stay inwardly focused, figuring out their problems.

The clearest analogy is the way our bodies respond to other environmental problems. Think about when your body is attacked by the flu virus. What happens? You get a fever, your body ratchets up the heat to try and fry the little buggers out of your system. And what do you know—you sleep weird, either more or less, and your eating habits change. Just like depression, the response to fever would appear, at first, to be an evolutionary disadvantage. But as Andrews points out, like fever, the down-regulated way our bodies and behaviors respond to depression could be "just another trade off" in the long line of ways we've adapted evolutionarily.

There are multiple kinds of depression—some that seem to stem from chemical imbalances or environmental stimuli. Even lack of sunlight can lead to seasonal affective disorder, which is usually referred to with the world's most convenient acronym, SAD. But the research points out that there are different depressive states, and Andrews for one would contend that not getting enough sunshine—which can adversely affect serotonin, a neurotransmitter that many researchers believe plays a role in regulating mood—is a *different* kind of depression.

THE STONE-SKIPPING TREATMENT PROGRAM

Whether it's fair or not, teachers are saddled with dealing with more and more students who have been diagnosed, or exhibit signs of, depression. One of the easiest ways to address this is to take them outdoors to play. Research aside, we all know from personal experience that getting out into the sunshine and air, seeing some green trees, and walking around a bit can usually disperse the gray cloud over our heads. But there may be a deeper reason to get students and kids outdoors more. It may be vital for them developing the analytical capabilities—to ruminate—on the complex problems facing them in their lives.

Remember, rumination helps you understand the nature of your problem, why the problem occurred, generates possible solutions, and evaluates those solutions. That progression is the basis of analytical thought, and by not giving children the chance to mope around the woods, kicking up leaves, idly skipping stones, or sitting glumly by the bank of a river watching the water flow, we may be robbing them not just of the opportunity to develop solutions to complex situations through fostering analytical thought—we may be taking away the opportunity for autonomous, therapeutic experience.

It seems that Thoreau knew this implicitly. After his brother died, he needed to get away—get into nature, out in the woods, and ruminate. The whole of *Walden* can be read as a treatise on how to *deal*. How to move through the world in a way that doesn't make you feel like a sell-out, or at least live a life that has happiness, fulfillment, and contentment as possibilities. Remember,

Thoreau was suffering. He was depressed and needed to find a way out of the melancholic miasma that surrounded him after his brother died. The path that led to his salvation headed off into the scrubby, unpopulated woods that surrounded Concord.

I love teaching and have spent the better part of twenty years working with students from preschool through college. I work predominantly with undergrads now, and many students have either expressed to me, or written about, their struggles with depression. I try to be as empathetic as possible, which isn't hard. I was just like them.

My mother died of a cerebral hemorrhage when I was seventeen years old. I was already at loose ends as a teenager. I did poorly in school and was somewhat of a troublemaker—and her death shook me to my roots. I spent the next few years pretending that it didn't happen, but the emotional effects were clear. Though there were times when I felt all right—working for Outward Bound for a while seemed to provide me with some solace—I had never really faced up to the reality of her death.

By the time I was twenty-one I was in a pretty sorry state. I'd dropped out of college, and worked as a dishwasher at a steakhouse in Los Angeles. I skipped on my rent all the time (much to the consternation of my roommates), had disastrous relationships, consumed vast oceans of alcohol, smoked, and generally acted like a complete jerk. I was depressed and began to have some pretty dark thoughts.

On a whim, I sold my truck, quit my job, and took the greyhound up to Monterey in Northern California. From there, I hitchhiked down the Pacific Coast Highway toward Big Sur. The coast of California around there—with redwood trees, sweeping vistas, and gorgeous, non-peopled beaches populated by massive elephant seals—is a mystical place. I went there in part because I'd read Henry Miller's *Big Sur and the Oranges of Hieronymus Bosch*, his memoir of almost two decades living in the area.

I didn't have much money, so I hiked up into canyons at night (likely trespassing), and pitched a little tent to sleep. By day I hiked around, hung out on the coast, bought food from camp stores and gas stations, and did a whole lot of nothing. I was by myself, for the most part. I was in the forest, outside. I was near the sea. I was ruminating.

I didn't have any transcendent moments of realization. I didn't all of a sudden become okay with my mom's death. I didn't feel particularly better, but as I look back now I'm pretty sure that the rumination I experienced there got me past some blockade—solved a complex problem—and allowed me to eventually buy a Greyhound ticket back to Los Angeles, where I soon began working at a Waldorf school and finding my love of teaching.

I imagine the parents of the students I teach at the expensive college I work at would be pretty angry if the advice I gave their kids to treat their depression was to sell everything they own and hitchhike the coast of Northern California. But that's not the real risk the students I have are facing in terms of their depression. Rumination happens most readily outside. But it also requires time and space to focus inwardly.

How are the students of today able to give themselves over to the necessary rumination required to solve complex problems if they're forever *connected*—always on their phones, swiping and clicking? Andrews noted that part of depression was the disconnectedness we feel—the way we draw away from others and into ourselves. If we truly want to teach the next generation of students, and as educators and parents we're also expected to deal with issues like depression, we need to find our way back to the kind of experiences that foster that deep, hard, solitary work of figuring out complex problems. Not everyone can head off into the woods like Thoreau to get over their brother's death, or to Big Sur like me. But one thing is for sure: if our children are distracted and constantly wired, we've removed rumination as an option.

I worried that this was just my own, anecdotal experience. So I put the question to Andrews. If rumination is part of the problem-solving process in depression—the what and the why—is it possible that the way children and college students live their lives now is creating a disconnect in that linear progression? To ruminate, we need solitude, time, and the chance to grapple with the complex problem. I asked him: do you think it's possible that the fact that kids are on their phones, playing video games, and trapped indoors in school may be a barrier to the process of rumination? Basically, doesn't rambling around the woods create a perfect scenario to engage in some rumination to work out those complex problems?

Andrews responded, "I think many features of modern life inhibit high quality rumination and the wisdom that would normally come from it."

And that, it seemed to me, was the most important part. What did Thoreau gain from his time at Walden Pond? Wisdom. It's a word I've never used in describing my teaching—that would be pretty egregiously pompous, I think—and I've always been scared to use it. Dumbledore and Gandalf are wise; kids who take my rhetoric course just learn to see through the bullshit of a campaign ad. But wisdom seemed possible, somehow, as a hoped-for goal. Perhaps the way to gain it is as simple as getting rid of our phones, and heading off, alone, into the woods—the antithesis of how schools are built and maintained.

CITY SICKERS

Schools are based in large part on the efficiency of factories. During the rise in Europe of what we would recognize as education during the eighteenth and nineteenth centuries, the factory model was deemed the most efficient means of educating as many children for the lowest cost possible. Put them in rows, indoors, and provide a conveyor belt curriculum so that learning between teacher and student can function at a low-cost proportional scale: 1–20, 1–30, or, in some university classrooms, 1–300 or so.

Furthermore, schools were based on the same kind of infrastructure that cities used. In order to fit all of the students into factory-like schools, buildings, and campuses, educational institutions had to be built in a certain way to maximize the use of space, control the flow of people, and impose efficiency and order on large groups of people.

The problem with this is that living in densely packed areas—cities—can give rise to anxiety. Researchers from the University of Heidelberg and McGill University in Montreal have shown that by situating ourselves in urban areas (the authors project that by 2050, almost 70 percent of the human race will be urban) we increased the likelihood of developing mental health issues. The authors conclude, "meta-analysis show that current city dwellers have a substantially increased risk for anxiety disorders (by 21%) and mood disorders (by 39%)."

One of the earliest people to pick up on this phenomenon was Carl Otto Westphal, a late nineteenth-century psychiatrist who noted in some of his patients a fear of particular spaces in urban environments such as very long bridges. Westphal called this fear *agoraphobia*, literally fear of spaces, not to be confused with the similar-sounding *agrophobia*, which means fear of open fields.

Freud added his own quirky take to the idea, suggesting that women in particular feared the open streets of the city as it would offer them freedom to express their repressed desire to become prostitutes—one of Freud's more spectacularly ridiculous claims, which is saying a lot. Regardless, what is clear is that when we constrain students to city-like environments, the results are less than perfect for learning. Kids and teachers get stressed. One of the easiest ways to alleviate some of the anxiety and stress is by heading out into the natural world, away from the institution.

The necessary efficiency of schools is its own validation. If we want to keep kids organized, safe, and relatively subdued, then creating institutions is a viable way to do so. But the question remains—why did we "institutionalize" schools? In my mind, institutionalization is a process that is inextricably bound with the indoor world, and thus it bears on our discussion of what would be possible if we started taking students out into the world. It may be helpful to figure out why we brought them indoors to begin with. What gains were made, compromises struck, and changes wrought by the adoption of hierarchies, rank, bureaucracy, and both philosophical and physical structures?

To answer this, we have to digress a bit. But first, it's important to remember that schools and education in anything resembling their current form are a relatively new creation. While there have been tutors, craft guilds, and all manner of structured teaching and learning for at least 4,000 years, our contemporary version of schools is only a few hundred years old, born mostly in western Europe through religious instruction married to notions of industrialized efficiency. And even if we include the training of scribes in the Fertile Crescent, we're still talking about a blip in the sweep of time modern humans have been around.

It's noteworthy here to briefly enter into our digression and ask what an educational institution *is*, and why it seems to require students to spend so much time indoors. We basically understand its functions and parts: school buildings, curricula, students, teachers. But as this book deals largely with the uncoupling of learning from the rigidity of institutionally imposed order, it may be helpful to try and understand what we talk about when we talk about institutions.

GET UP, STAND UP

As a word, at its etymological core, the word "institution" comes from the word "stand." Or, more precisely, from many old words that mean "stand," Old English *stangan*, Old High German *stantan*, and so on through various Latin cognates; *stare, stet, stand, stare*. But one of the more curious layers in the onion-y history of the word "institution" is its relation to the word "status" and "statesman" as well as "statistics"—the last word should sound familiar to anyone sitting in meetings talking about "targets" or "retention."

But in terms of its closest cousins, "institution" comes from the Latin *instituere*, to place in or upon. And here's where we get to an interesting piece of the profile of institutions. The Latin *instare* is also closely related, and means, according to Eric Partridge's book on the history of English words *Origins*, "to stand in or over against, hence to be menacing or urgent or imminent."

It's really just an intellectual exercise, and of course the word "institution" is only just that—a word. But it's helpful to think about the word in its etymological complexity simply for the fact that institutions such as schools, businesses, governments, hospitals, and so forth control so much of our lives. Its nuances should be made known, and in looking at the various corollaries and cognates of "institution" we can see that within its etymology is the very notion of rigid hierarchy—something that outdoor education works overtly against. The very core purpose of institutions—to regulate and control—are eroded out in the natural world, and replaced by a more diverse web of personal autonomy, collaboration, and agency.

BEING WELL

There is a nascent movement—particularly in higher education—of creating spaces for students focused on wellness and health. Most notably, the University of Vermont has developed entire dorms that support wellness through meditation, access to gyms, personal trainers, and, rather inexplicably, free Apple watches. The aim of programs like this is simple: instituting healthy lifestyles in students when they enter college can increase student performance, improve retention, and reduce the emphasis on punishing unhealthy choices (drugs, binge drinking) and replace it with positive alternatives. Behind this transition is a central tenet: to *learn* well one must *feel* well.

Being outdoors increases students' well-being. It is beneficial from both a physiological and psychological perspective. In a way, it has created positive institutional responses to the negative effects of being at an institution. For most teachers and schools, however, the ability to create massive, programmatic change similar to the University of Vermont runs into some pretty tough obstacles; budgets, time, expertise. However, taking students to outdoor environments—for long periods of time given over to explore, play, and ramble—could do some of the same work. This fee-form engagement with unstructured nature provides benefits that could change the classroom for the better. And the only barrier is an unconscious bias against the outdoors.

Chapter 4

The Outdoor Body

In my late thirties I began to experience a number of health problems. They were symptomatic of some larger, underlying chronic cause, but I had trouble identifying what, exactly, was wrong with me. I began to notice swelling in my abdomen. My skin was no longer as elastic and pliable—it seemed to have grown thin as though from a deficiency of some kind. My vision wasn't as acute as it had been, so I had to get reading glasses. My back hurt. When I drank alcohol, I was sick the next day, sometimes for two days, beyond what I considered a normal amount of fuzziness after a night on the town. My overall drive and energy just dropped, and my hair began to thin. I felt, most of the time, like I was winded and tired and worn out.

My concern reached its peak when I was walking my dog one day and slipped on a bit of ice—normally, my balance is pretty good and it wouldn't have affected me. In this case, though, I was unable to catch my balance and toppled over. I searched the internet, asked friends, and questioned medical professionals. Soon, the cause of my illness, my decline, became clear.

I was getting older.

This was, of course, horrifying. I mean me—older? Not a chance. I am youth incarnate, as full of piss and vinegar as Peter Pan. There was just no way—*no way*—I was reaching middle age.

And yet I was. As I hit my forties I was a full fifteen pounds heavier than I had been my whole life. I was slower and more cautious in my movements. The inexorable decline of my physical self was mirrored by what felt like an atrophied imagination—even my thoughts seemed frail and wizened with age.

It couldn't have come at a worse time. I was finally happy in a job I loved, teaching writing at a small New England college. My kids were both healthy and happy. I was working on a number of writing projects, some of

49

which—miracle among miracles—saw the light of day. My full-time position offered financial stability, medical benefits, and a clean, comfy office with hardwood floors. I even had an ergonomic office chair. I had access to two different gyms as part of my employment. I ran about three or four miles at least a few times a week. And yet, despite all of these advantages, my body felt shitty and lumpy and like it was falling apart.

I love teaching, reading, and writing, and, despite my love of the outdoors, I end up spending a good deal of time inside, getting work done, albeit frustrated and pining for pines. This incongruity in my temperament has been the leading cause of my restlessness my whole life—and possibly part of the reason my body was no longer, um, as *taut* as I'd like.

My own physical struggles are hardly unique. The idea of spending an hour or so, a couple of times a week, to stay in shape, is central to America's health culture. And while clearly exercise is a valuable pursuit, the way we've adapted our physical movement to our modern lives is not consistent with the way our bodies evolved to move. Sudden bursts of movement and exercise interspersed in a week that contains massive stretches of hours sitting isn't optimum. A day spent outdoors, navigating the natural physical challenges presented by unstructured nature, is more in keeping with how our bodies respond to exercise. Spending all day moving about in natural environments regulates our metabolism, keeps our muscles and bones strong and healthy, sharpens our vestibular system (balance), and may have other benefits, including keeping parts of our bodies other than our waistlines healthy and robust.

Around the time I turned forty I got my first pair of reading glasses. Over the weeks and months leading up to that moment, my face had become progressively more scrunched when I propped up a book at night to read; the page inched closer and closer to the tip of my nose as I tried to make out the fuzzy shapes of the letters on the page. "You should see your face!" Cindy would say laughingly as I struggled to bring the words into focus. Eyes squinted, brow furrowed, I fought against my weakening eyesight to little avail. I now bring my glasses everywhere since I can't work without them.

SEEING IS BELIEVING

I am part of what may be a global pandemic of rapidly deteriorating eyesight. According to a slew of research from both U.S. and Asian Universities, myopia is on the rise the world over, but particularly in places like China and Korea, and especially in adolescents and people in their twenties. How bad is it? According to a 2015 article in *Nature*, shortsightedness affected between 10 and 20 percent of China's population sixty years ago; now it's a full *90 percent*. And for nineteen-year-old males in Seoul, Korea, there's over a 96 percent chance they're shortsighted.

One of the prevailing myths has always been that lots of reading leads to wearing glasses, hence the iconic caricature of the bespectacled bookworm. One would think that too many days spent absorbed in novels on the couch would eventually lead to glasses due to the small size of the print in books. However, the research paints a significantly different picture of the causes of chronic vision impairment. In fact, there appears *not* to be a simple, one-way, direct relationship between traditional book reading and poor eyesight. The research is teasing out a more nuanced story to explain why so many individuals across the world are experiencing deteriorating vision.

It comes down to too much time spent indoors.

Yes, screens play a role as well. But the fact is most screens are indoors—while it is possible for individuals to stare at smartphones as they navigate the city sidewalks, anecdotal evidence would suggest it's unwise; the internet is replete with viral videos of people texting and then walking into fountains, walls, and, in one particularly memorable post, running into a bear rummaging through garbage in an alley.

The way the human eye functions outdoors, it turns out, is different from how they operate indoors. Research suggests that it comes down to light and distance—and our eyes are supremely adapted to the kind of light, and kind of distances, that are experienced outdoors. The people with the best eyesight in the world are Australian Aborigines, the last large-scale hunter-gatherer society to be dismantled through colonization, and thus one of the few remaining groups on the planet with valid ties to their hunter-gatherer pasts. Professor Hugh Taylor of the University of Melbourne has documented Aboriginal "super sight" through his research, and it appears that a lifetime spent in the bush, tracking animals and traversing terrain, is just the sort of lifestyle that contributes to healthy eyesight.

But I had spent tons of time outside over the last two decades—why was this happening to me? Since the rise of the internet, I'd spent more and more time indoors hunched in front of a screen. I got my first email address around 2003 at the age of twenty-nine. (I avoided it as long as I could.) And since that time I've spent more and more time in my professional and personal life using the screen to get things done, entertain myself, escape from reality, and even exercise, courtesy of Shaun T. and Jillian Michaels. Was I, too, like the students in places like Korea and China suffering from the twenty-first century's first techno-affliction: chronic debilitating vision deterioration brought on by indoor living?

Working or spending time indoors doesn't directly correlate to impaired vision necessarily. Eyesight can begin to deteriorate for the same reason that people can't run as fast, or jump as high, as time passes: age. Or, it could be partially inherited. Many vision impairments such as shortsightedness are genetic. But the current shift that the modern world has imposed on a previously outdoor, landscape-traversing species is abrupt, and modern science is only recently beginning to examine the correlation between eyesight and large amounts of time spent indoors looking at screens.

While the Australian Aborigines are unique, research suggests that being outdoors—particularly for children—is the best way to preserve eyesight and hold off the development of shortsightedness. The human eye evolved to be able to manipulate small things with incredible accuracy—humans can pluck fleas off a dog—but also for taking in wide swaths of terrain. The health of the eye depends, at least in part, on the balance between these two activities. Until very recently on an evolutionary timescale, the human eye was perfectly accustomed to absorbing the ongoing scene around a village, following a track through the bush, or looking for vultures circling around as they searched for prey. Eyes are adept at focusing on a loved-one's face and processing that recognition, and well attuned to capture details in the environment. But most of the time, in evolutionary terms, people looked at things outside, in the full light of day.

Things have changed. Now, in the digitized world, whether in Lagos, Laos, or Los Angeles, many humans spend an inordinate amount of time in front of screens. Doing so forces the eye to follow a blinking cursor less than a centimeter high as it blips across the field of vision. People have gone from looking at the very large world around them to looking at a very small screen in less than a century. Individuals in the modern world spend a tremendous amount of time at computers, indoors, and the effects of this lifestyle are very possibly responsible for the current trend in deteriorating eyesight, especially in youth.

Herein lies the traditional dilemma faced by educators—the gains to be made by indoor reading, writing, and learning versus the advantages of outdoor experiences. But this dualistic view is overly simplistic. It is not an either/or problem, but rather one in which the complexity of learning and the goals of education need to take into account mind–body dynamics and the intellectual and physical well-being of students.

If the studies of those students from places like Seoul and Guangzhou are any indication, humans have arrived at a time when the very tools and learning experiences that are pressed into service in the name of educating children are actually doing them harm—at the very least to their eyesight. This is perhaps a small price to pay in exchange for participation in the rewards of the technocracy that pervades the economic narrative of the current global culture. But if this is accepted as inevitable, what chain of events has been ushered in? Anemic bodies, weakened skeletons. Will humans become like the future humans depicted in Pixar's *WALL-E*, floating around on screen-laden easy chairs, slurping food through straws searching for the next distraction while their body parts morph into something resembling soft, fungal lobes? This is an issue separate from the way in which media-saturated cultural "norms" have twisted body-image expectations. This is an issue that addresses the very basic health of children and what role education plays in it.

HYPOTHERMIC HIGH ACHIEVERS

Some sobering statistics, courtesy of the U.S. Department of Health and Human Services, are vital in identifying what the cost in terms of health is that students pay by participating in traditional, indoor education experiences. One-third of children aged six to nineteen are overweight or obese. One in six of that age group is considered medically obese. One in six. That's scary. What's scarier is that those kids grow up to be adults, of whom more than two out of three are considered overweight or obese. That's over 66 percent of adults carrying around extra weight. Some diseases that result from chronic obesity are type 2 diabetes, heart disease, and liver problems. Obesity in children has been called an epidemic, and it is. How can kids learn—explore the world, feel good about themselves, and engage fully in mind–body learning—when they can barely move?

This issue closely parallels fat-shaming but has the important distinction of being related to medically assessable health rather than culturally dictated morphology. Body type, lifestyle, and physiology are one thing. It is not education's job to "norm" people with larger than "normal" body mass indexes, or institute some Hollywood-inspired, fascistic regime where all students need to look good in spandex. Here in the United States, the general conception of body types, and the way women in particular are viewed through dominant media, are dangerously out of step with realistic bodies. But it's important to note that the challenges facing education is not body-type or lifestyle choices in adults; the challenges lie in the relationship between the fact that traditional schooling keeps kids inside all day, what that does to their metabolic rates and bodies, and how it affects their overall health.

Brown adipose tissue—or BAT—is a specific kind of fat that differs from the types of cells normally considered "fat" cells. Brown fat plays a specific role in dissipating energy to make sure body temperature stays constant—something called thermogenesis. Thermogenesis is the process whereby body temperature is maintained despite what the environmental temperature is—whether it's a chilly 32 degrees Fahrenheit or a blistering 90, the body regulates itself to maintain a temperature somewhere in the neighborhood of 98.6. It's why humans can live in places like Ottawa and Stockholm but most reptiles can't. They don't have the same thermogenesis engines humans do.

Of course, if things get too cold the human body can get hypothermic; too hot and the result is heat exhaustion. However, there's a substantially wide range of temperatures where humans can exist. BAT has other properties as well: glucose uptake, spurring metabolism, and regulating insulin sensitivity. Children have lots of BAT, but recently researchers have discovered that adults have it as well, primarily in the neck, around the collarbones, and along the spine. One of the ways to fire up all those good things about BAT—its ability to burn fatty acids, regulate metabolism, balance insulin—is by going outside when it's cold.

The research on BAT and its resultant effect on metabolism strongly suggest that exposing people to cold ramps up the way BAT can help humans maintain an appropriate balance between energy intake and energy expenditure. Obesity is an imbalance in this exact equation—too much fuel in and not enough fuel burned.

In a study from *Cell Press* titled "Brown fat fuel utilization and thermogenesis," the authors state, "two studies have demonstrated that cold acclimation in humans, after repeated daily cold-exposure, results in an increase in BAT activity with a surge in energy expenditure." In fact, the study goes on to state that when we introduce bodies to cold environments, the amount of glucose that muscles consumed increased twelve times.

All of this brings about the question: what has an indoor lifestyle done to the body's ability to metabolize in such a way to efficiently burn fuel? Has it made humans unhealthy by not forcing metabolism to compensate for low temperatures? Students are inside for most of their time in school. Their bodies' natural mechanisms for regulating temperature aren't engaged by their environment, depriving them of the benefits of metabolic processes that keep their bodies healthy.

Another study from the same publication, this one led by a researcher from the Netherlands with the fun-to-say name of Wouter van Marken Lichtenbelt (try it three times fast, I dare you), states the argument most clearly thus:

> In the past century several dramatic changes in the daily living circumstances in Western civilization have occurred, affecting health. For example, we are much better able to control our ambient temperature. Consequently, we cool and heat our dwellings for maximal comfort while minimizing our body energy expenditure necessary to control body temperature.

In a nutshell, bodies don't have to work as hard to stay warm, and the result is that the excess fuel normally designated to staying warm gets converted to fat. The study goes on to state that most people in the western world spend some 90 percent of the time indoors in temperature-controlled environments. Most buildings are around 65 to 75 degrees—a variation of only 10 degrees.

The study points out that not only does this homoeothermic environment affect health, but energy consumption—usually in the form of fossil fuels—rockets skyward.

Every winter it seems like there's a news story about how mothers in Denmark leave their babies in strollers outside during the winter while they drink coffee in cafes. While it's a cute story, the basis of the tradition may go as deep as brown adipose tissue. When students are denied time outdoors, it limits more than their imaginations. The danger is greater than taking away the chance for them to develop balance, strong muscles and bones, and cooperative, collaborative games. On a very basic level, schools often injure their health by not allowing student bodies' natural metabolic functions to act in the way they've evolved to act. The key to all this is the way that bodies evolved to deal with temperature. Humans are quite adept at surviving and thriving in a variety of temperatures. There's only a few other mammals that can exist at all the different temperatures that we can.

The downside is clear: kids are gaining weight, running the risk of diabetes, and atrophying important metabolic processes by being indoors too much. And the place they spend all day, five days a week, some 180 days a year? School. If education's goal is to raise *healthy*, smart, engaged citizens, it fails when the students are kept indoors all day.

GUIDING LIGHT

While humans don't have the same relation to sunlight as plants, depending on it for metabolizing food through photosynthesis, it's hard not to surmise that being outdoors in fresh air and sunlight gives people a boost—energizing their very souls. And while this may sound like the sort of annoying boosterism of a Vermont mountain hippie (guilty as charged), it's also backed by some pretty substantial research.

Research from the *Journal of Environmental Psychology* points to time outdoors as having "vitalizing effects." Simply put, the term "vitality" in psychological parlance means having both mental and physical energy. Feeling good, charged up, and ready to go. The link between being outdoors in nature and this vital feeling of energy is key because not only do individuals in nature feel a burst of energy, but they also reconfigure their brains and have better stress response mechanisms. Basically, people in these natural, outdoor environments in the studies exhibit better coping strategies for stress, and also have a greater overall level of well-being and health. But other benefits to spending time outdoors are even more dynamic. Higher levels of vitality also increase the body's defense systems, and humans become less prone to viral and environmental stressors the more time they spend outside. They get sick less often.

SHUT UP, DESCARTES!

The fundamental discrepancy in education is that there is *education* and there is *physical education*. This duality hearkens back to the age-old Cartesian mind–body divide, which neuroscience, psychology, and physiological research has largely debunked—or at least reframed—over the past 100 years. Outdoor learning incorporates both the mind and body into experience, creating a holistic approach that engenders deeper understanding, more permanent and accessible memories, and a stronger body to support further investigation. In denying children access to large amounts of playtime outdoors, schools risk more than not providing students with ample time to play; it undermines the very process of learning itself, rooted in the bodily experience of personal development.

Experiential learning is holistic. It educates the mind and body, but also teaches interpersonal skills, instructs us in ethics, increases the capacity for grit, and fosters compassion and empathy. Personal development is the unavoidable dividend of experiential education, as is the opportunity for genuine self-reflection. Unlike more narrow ways of learning, outdoor education has both the cultivation of abstract reasoning and the practical application of skills and abilities. Much of this comes from the inherently physical nature of being outdoors.

There is such an emphasis placed on abstract thinking in absentia of experience in school that learning can seem divorced from reality for many students—they aren't able to integrate it into their own concept of themselves and the world because they have no actual, bodily experience with which to process the learning. Interestingly, it is often the intellectual projects that are the most clearly derived from experience versus pure reasoning—that are situated as much in the body as in the mind. Take writing a book, for example. It's a misnomer that writers sit down, pen in hand, and a book pours forth, direct from the honeyed celestial realms of imagination. I wish. Most writers spend far more time preparing for writing: finding sources of information and inspiration; engaging in research that could involve direct experience, travel, interviews, or experimentation. There's a fair amount of hand-wringing and talking to oneself. Staring vacantly out windows is also an essential component, as is walking the dog.

And then, there is life to be lived; jobs, family, kids, friends, and the (to me) frustrating confinement of institutional demands. Standing in line at the grocery store. Filling out school registration packets. Forever going online, switching smaller and smaller piles of money between savings and checking accounts to cover the monthly bills. Fixing leaky faucets. Not very sexy. The writing only comes months, or years, after all the preliminary experiences have been dumped into the pot to be simmered down into a readable chunk of prose.

Words and ideas take up residence in the body before they're on the page. They're chewed up and spit out. Digested. Rejected. In some traditions within Judaism, students in Hebrew School are asked to read the *Torah* standing, even rocking from foot to foot, to better incorporate (a word which literally means "take into the body") the meaning and import of the text. The body is the medium through which learning manifests itself, and the way in which it occurs is through direct, physical experience. This phenomenon has been widely studied within embodied cognition, and what it boils down to is that thinking as we know it is an embodied, experientially based process.

Even the kind of thinking that—at cursory first glance—seems purely abstract and intellectual is based on those experiences. By adopting a curriculum that places outdoor experiences in the unstructured, outdoor world center stage, schools would be frontloading the kind of personal reference points needed for students to process the lessons they've learned.

The tradition of *learning by doing* goes by many names; in the modern context, it's often referred to as place-based learning, expeditionary learning, environmental education, experiential learning. While there are many attributes to the various forms of outdoor education, particular attention must be paid to *unstructured outdoor experiences in natural environments* and how they relate to learning. This is exclusive of the benefits of organized environmental education programs that take place outdoors, or the sort of field work associated with studying natural resource management. Both those examples are worthy of their own studies, and there has been plenty of work done evaluating the benefit of those types of programs.

While there are numerous similarities, the benefit to be derived from children (and adults!) spending large amounts of time in natural environments: woods, mountains, deserts, or watery places like rivers, lakes, and oceans cannot be underestimated. Places where the intermediary influence of institutionalized pedagogy is nonexistent, and a more organic, holistic approach to learning and human development arises in harmony with the environment itself. The key to these benefits are in the very bodily nature of the learning. While it seems a simplification, it's not: when students' bodies are outside, they incorporate their learning in a more dynamic, lasting fashion than when they're indoors.

What happens when we allow children and students to be in open, natural environments and experience them through *the framework of self and each other* rather than through some prescribed pedagogical lens? It is in these circumstances that the combination of body–mind interactions reaches their zenith, in this interstitial space between organized educational activities and total chaos—a place where physical, emotional, and intellectual development is cultivated and the capacity is developed for empathy and imagination.

One of the obstacles faced by outdoor education is the intangibility of the results. Many institutions of higher learning, in order to evaluate student progress in traditional academic terms, have developed a kind of digital portfolio of student work to be used to assess them as well as give students a chunk of work that spans their collegiate experience so they can reflect on their own learning—likely a helpful tool in calculating the development of critical thinking and problem solving in a narrow, indoor-oriented sense. But this movement toward the digital archiving of student performance also comes from a place where institutions denote improvement through the categorical assessment of traditional academic skills: analysis, conscientiousness, and critical thinking. While these are excellent skills to have, the narrowness of the current manner of evaluating student performance focuses only on the ability to reflect the attainment or mastery of codified skills; but there are other developmental achievements that don't receive the same attention. Contemplation as opposed to critical thinking, as an example. The other non-assessed realm is the way students are "in touch" with their bodies. How grounded are they within their physicality? This is separate from athletic ability. It is an understanding of their physicality, and the way in which the body moves through space. Allowing students time outside to stretch and strengthen their bodies doesn't distract them from learning; it increases the "uptake" of new ideas, concepts, and skills in a way no other type of experience is able to.

Developing the ability in students to assign meaning to their lives; to define a narrative based not on ticking off boxes or prescribed educational achievement, but one based on the development of self, and the creation of a self-mythology that provides agency and empowerment should be a central component of education. Schools should be fostering the skill required to stop and notice things—to be mindful of the present, themselves, and others. These abilities are rooted in the body—and in getting the body outdoors senses like balance, movement, and sight engage kinesthetic learning.

GETTING DOWN WITH YOUR MINDFUL SELF

Lately it's been a good thing to be in the mindfulness business. Clad in quasi-Buddhist ideologies and New Age-y feel-goodism, mindfulness as a practice is everywhere, from yoga studios to therapy offices. And while much of the conversation about mindfulness is a rather hollow, hipster-fueled exercise in silliness, at its core it remains a central tenet of many religions in the world, and a complex and demanding psychological practice.

In essence, mindfulness seeks to expand consciousness by focusing on the here and now. In order to achieve mindfulness, one meditates and focuses only on breathing, trying to recognize but quell the annoying diatribe of the nagging inner voice, as one example of a diverse range of methodologies.

Mindfulness practices include walking silently around the room, eating raisins one by one—there is a multitude of ways to try and engage in an experience that allows the practitioner to be intimately aware of the body. One of the ways that has gained a certain amount of traction of late is by going outdoors. But certainly one of the keys of mindfulness is the grounding of the self in the body, and developing an awareness of the state of our physical being.

By infusing outdoor experiences in the way in which we educate children, opportunities are provided to practice mindfulness. Mindfulness has been used successfully in a variety of therapeutic scenarios and been somewhat useful in treating depression, anxiety, and some learning disorders. Experiential education—particularly in rugged, unstructured landscapes—practically *demands* mindfulness. Tired and stumbling, as they shuffle down the mountain toward the end of the day, it's all students can do to focus on not tripping over the bricolage of tree roots and stubbornly upright rocks in their path. The brain achieves a rather blank state as tired hikers narrow their perception to the path in front with no thoughts in their heads save the occasional prayer for pizza and ice cream.

Mindfulness—the ability to be present in the moment and in touch with the senses—despite the overwhelming amount of commercialization it has experienced over the past few decades—is central to learning. Being outdoors facilitates the experience of *noticing what you notice*, one of the ways that mindfulness gets us to narrow perception but at the same time open senses to the surroundings. The benefit of dialing in the state of the body goes beyond calming and meditative mindsets—it introduces techniques that underlie central educational skills like concentration, focus, and will power.

Ajahn Buddhadasa was a twentieth-century Thai Buddhist philosopher and ascetic who called this "natural samadhi"—the ability to be contemplative and present in the outdoors. Buddhadasa practiced his stripped-down form of Buddhist mindfulness in a small tract of forest near his village in Thailand. From Buddhadasa and those like him it's possible to draw a line to the modern experience of the outdoors, which is usually replete with GPS, selfies, and lots of chattering banter among the hiking party. All lovely things—indeed, I've been known to indulge in a mountain top selfie myself—but there is this other side of experiential education in nature, where the senses are allowed to develop in ways that don't normally have the opportunity to expand during hectic school days. While education seems comfortable with the idea of providing younger children with the chance to bodily experience nature, as they progress through the grades, they get less time outside, fewer opportunities to experience mindfulness, and less experience sensing their own bodies' existence in the world.

By the time students get to college, it is as though their bodies no longer exist. The default mode of teaching is indoors and sedentary. Schools leave behind the holistic approach introduced in kindergarten—outside playtime and instructor-led social collaboration—in favor of ever narrowing skill sets defined largely by the economic imperatives of the job market. This is unfortunate on multiple levels. By the college years, the population of students also experience an uptick in unhealthy habits; sleep deprivation, poor nutrition, and lack of exercise. An educational approach that centralized outdoor experiences would mitigate some of the negative effects of weight gain known as "the freshman 15" that many college students experience.

Outdoor education is the realest of the real of all learning experiences. There's no place to hide—both teacher and student are exposed. Antipathies come to light; vulnerabilities are on display. Quite literally, *who we are* is what comes to matter most.

Recently, the simplicity of attempting a pedagogical approach that incorporates this understanding of the role of the physical body in learning was elucidated in an article by Del Doughty, a professor and dean at Huntington University. In the essay, Doughty extols the virtues of the "walking meeting," or even a "walking class." Sick of being indoors all day, Doughty tells his students to read up on their work and get ready to walk and talk. They do, and he extends the lesson to both his advisees and classes in general. The result? Experiential education.

It's not some mysterious, difficult-to-grasp concept. Getting students out into the open air, moving their bodies, and engaging with their environment changed things for Doughty. He sought the solution as a way to shake off the frustration and inertia of a long day in the office, and to capitalize on nice weather, but the benefits of engaging in direct, physical experience were clear:

> Walking with students was a break from the usual, it kept things fresh, it built rapport. In terms of teaching dynamics, I liked it, because when I walked side by side with someone, it diminished or removed many of those obstacles that stand in the way of learning. There were no podiums, screens, clunky technologies, classroom management protocols. We talked back and forth, and we listened to each other as walkers do. Sometimes we would bring a book or an article, and sometimes we would stop and search for a passage that came up in the course of our conversation. We were literally on equal footing out there.

This ethos—a face-to-face, less structured interaction that occurs in a natural, organic fashion—is part of a growing understanding within the broader community of researchers, writers, and teachers who are exploring just what, exactly, has gone wrong with our schools. Anthropologist Susan Blum contrasts these two types of learning—organic, naturally collaborative and non-standards based with the hierarchical, codified learning—in her book *I Love Learning, I Hate School: An Anthropology of College*.

Blum refers to learning outside of school, such as the experiences that help us develop our sense of self, community, and environment that we experience in natural settings, as "learning in the wild," and refers to traditional learning on a college campus as "learning in the cage." This idea that learning can happen in these sorts of challenging environments is something that schools have, by and large, lost sight of. The very structures put in place in schools can often limit learning, rather than promote it. The easiest, most direct way to escape from "the cage" is to go outdoors, into natural settings, and let students' natural curiosity take the lead.

Chapter 5

Reading the Wild

I have no idea how I found the book, nor why it was there. The library of the college where I work is small, but the stacks are excellently curated. In terms of the courses we teach, there are pretty great materials available. I was down in the basement, scuttling along browsing through the books, and I found a particular volume that seemed a bit out of place. The book was *The Vagabond in Literature*, by an English writer named Arthur Rickett. The book was slim and so old the pages had turned a deep, orangey-yellow. It seemed an odd book—it had a narrow, rather irrelevant scope. And yet, as is the case with many books we stumble on, it lit a fire for me in terms of thinking about the relationship between reading, the outdoors, and teaching.

Rickett is largely absent from the digital archives of the web. He wrote a few literature studies in the early twentieth century. But this book of Rickett's grabbed me right away. While 100 years old, it firmly linked what to my mind are two spheres: the wilderness of the world and the wilderness of our imagination.

Rickett wrote the book as a commentary on some British writers (Hazlitt, De Quincey, and Robert Louis Stevenson) as well as a couple of Americans (Thoreau and Whitman) and the way their love of the wild transmuted itself into their writing:

> There are some men born with a vagrant strain in the blood, an insatiable inquisitiveness about the world beyond their doors. Natural revolutionaries they, with an ingrained distaste for the routine of ordinary life and the conventions of civilization.

Rickett notes in his book that the idea of exploring the wilderness, for some of these writers, may in fact be only metaphoric, but that hardly matters, as what interests Rickett is the shared love these writers have of untrammeled spaces—be they woodsy or those of ideas. "Sometimes, the vagabond is a physical, sometimes only an intellectual wanderer; but in any case there is about him something of the primal wildness of the woods and hills."

Rickett's book—to his credit—steers clear of the sort of woozy, metaphysical stuff writers can succumb to when waxing philosophic about nature and art. Because while these writers experienced "an intense joy in the open air," Rickett also places them within the more practical confines of secularity and modernity: "There is nothing mystical or abstract about it," the forgotten writer tells us, "it is direct, personal, intimate."

This is a good place to begin to look at how literature—especially literature about the outdoors—inspires exploration and, unfortunately, exploitation of the outdoors itself.

LEARNING IS ROOTED IN BOOKS

Before we all started gamboling about the digital landscape like a bunch of mindless dopamine-addicted leprechauns tweeting and tagging and sharing in a pixelated trance, and thus forced education to follow suit by offering learning that's described as "high impact" and "technologically relevant" and basically sold our souls to software companies in Silicon Valley, we mostly used books to teach about ideas and ethics and history and the idea of self. By the way, I'm not pointing fingers here. As I write this chapter, it's only 10:13 a.m. and I've already checked Twitter three times.

While many exorbitantly expensive private colleges with endowments as big as the GDP of Portugal continue to teach out of books within the safety of their ivy-encased campuses, most schools have felt in various degrees of intensity the tectonic shift in education toward learning that is less concerned with books. However, if there is any repository worth diving into to help figure out where we stand as educators when it comes to outdoor experiences and their connection to learning, books are a good place to start. After all, much of our educational and cultural history is bound up in stories and novels—while being rapidly superseded by the digital medium they are still, arguably, foundational to western thought. Maybe not for long, but at least for now.

Robinson Crusoe is one of the most fundamental adventure stories in English literature. So deeply embedded in our culture is it that it's hard to look at any story of an individual in nature and not be reminded of Daniel Defoe's 1719 masterpiece. It is believed that Defoe based his fictional account, at least in part, on the real-life travails of Alexander Selkirk, a Scottish sailor who spent four years alone on an island until he was rescued in 1709.

Defoe's tale of a middle-class Englishman living for over twenty years on a deserted island is one of the books that is so deeply intertwined in the collective consciousness that I've always claimed to have read it, despite the fact that I wasn't sure if I actually had read it, or just knew the tale so well through its prevalence in culture that I could pull off pretending to know it. It is true—in part—that I've read *Robinson Crusoe*. When I was a kid my parents got me a picture book version. I remember reading and rereading it, totally absorbed in the story of an Englishman trapped on a tropical island, surviving only on his wits and what he could salvage from the wreck of his ship. The pages were filled with great illustrations by N. C. Wyeth, pictures of Crusoe strolling about with goatskin knickers under a goatskin umbrella.

The book fired in me a desire for adventure, resourcefulness, and exploration, and specifically the sorts of adventures and requirements for ingenuity that would be required on a deserted island. Years later, when I got to camp on an uninhabited island in the Florida Keys after sailing there with Outward Bound in an old wood-hulled, canvas-sailed boat, I felt as if my dream had come true.

Children's literature is rife with stories of people (and sometimes animals) stranded on deserted islands. *The Cay*, by Theodore Taylor, is a fantastic kid's novel from the latter half of the twentieth century about a blind boy, Phillip, and an elderly black man, Timothy, stranded on a small, narrow island together. Set in the World War II era, the novel is rich ground for discussion, as Phillip displays deep prejudice against Timothy but due to his recent blindness (he's struck in the head and loses his sight shortly after the ship he's sailing on is torpedoed) must depend on the old man to survive. In confronting his infirmity and helpless he also confronts his racist beliefs—both literal and psychological blindness are tested within the sandy confines of the island.

In *Hatchet*, a novel by Gary Paulsen, a young boy is forced to survive in the Canadian wilderness with only the eponymous tool to help him. *Island of the Blue Dolphins* by Scott O'Dell, *Abel's Island* by William Steig, the novel *The Black Stallion*—even *Treasure Island* by Robert Louis Stevenson is tangentially about a marooned sailor, Ben Gunn, on a deserted island.

I read these books as a kid with voracious abandon, and have since taught some of them to students. I find that since they reduce the plane of action usually to one or two characters within a confined, limited space, they're so elegant in their presentation of basic human concerns (food, water, shelter), but also of the thornier, more difficult-to-nail-down stuff like identity, individualism, and our relationship with unbounded nature. They are—or were, for me—an essential building block in the way I conceptualized nature as an idea as a kid. Something to be survived, overcome, and defeated. It was an antagonist to be battled, to be subdued. All of these "islandic" books reduce the plot—and the central idea—to an elemental struggle of opposites. Man versus Nature.

Robinson Crusoe is arguably the forefather of all these stories. The struggles Crusoe experiences provide the template for much of what comes after in literature, story, and cultural narrative about the way we relate to the wild, uninhabited corners of the world, and thus feeds our deeply held convictions about our relationship with nature.

I sat down to read the original text of *Robinson Crusoe* recently. I have to admit, though while not exactly a ripping yarn, I was pretty entertained. I've always been a fan of nouns, and thus I like stories in which *things* are in the forefront more than *ideas*. And, as Virginia Woolf points out in a critical essay she wrote concerning Robinson Crusoe, "There are no sunsets and no sunrises; there is no solitude and no soul. There is, on the contrary, staring us full in the face nothing but a large earthenware pot."

The story of Robinson Crusoe's adventures is very much a book of stuff. Crusoe, as narrator, details everything he salvages from the wreck of his ship before it is swept away by a storm. Bread, rice, three "Dutch cheeses," five pieces of "dry'd Goat's flesh," two good fowling pieces, two pistols, powder horns, two "old rusty swords," two saws, an ax, and a hammer. The list goes on and on. Defoe writes endlessly about Crusoe's efforts to get an abominably heavy roll of sheet lead off the wreck and onto his little homemade raft to be floated across the surf to the island. There are entire sections of the novel where—as other writers have pointed out—Crusoe's labor is like an ant's, a sort of mindless toil and antic industriousness fills the pages.

Once on the island, Crusoe begins constructing a home for himself: part cave, part tent, and part fort. He is—from the beginning of the novel to the end—afraid of just about everything. Wild animals, black people, storms, lightening—Crusoe is a man besieged by the world around him (so he thinks) and believes the world is full of evil intent. We are given page after page of his descriptions of the defensive wall he builds around his little home—sharpened sticks and only a ladder to get over it. A veritable fortress.

Earlier in the story, as Crusoe sails south along the coast of Africa on a different voyage, we get a glimpse of how the middle-class tradesman Crusoe thinks of nature: "as soon as it was quite dark we heard such Dreadful Noises of the Barking, Roaring, and Howling of Wild Creatures . . . Xury was dreadfully frighted, and indeed so was I too."

It's not just "Creatures" Crusoe fears; the inhabitants of the African coast are clearly put into the same category as the wild beasts:

> There was no going on Shoar for us in the Night upon that Coast, and how to Venture on Shoar in the Day was another Question too; for to have fallen into the Hands of any of the Savages had been as bad as to have fallen into the Hands of Lyons and Tygers.

The description is standard colonial fare; equating indigenous populations with animals was a consistent theme in European exploration. Crusoe does eventually meet some of the "savages," who give him fresh water and food and are not at all violent—though that does little to change Crusoe's opinion toward other races.

Crusoe's fear defines him, and also defines his view of the natural world around him. Robinson Crusoe's very attitude toward nature is that it must be subdued, under his command, exploited, controlled, and, above all, feared. This fear and desire to conquer and control nature extends to "savages" who Crusoe clearly sees as not part of the human race, but part of the threatening world around him.

Even when he finds no savage creatures on the island, Crusoe still lives in fear, trying to recreate an English manor on his island, growing crops, making pottery, and praying with his Bible. Crusoe's notion of a nature walk is to shoot first and ask questions later.

Defoe was writing during the age of slavery. In fact, the reason the fictitious Crusoe gets marooned in the first place is that he's signed on to a slave-raiding ship bound for Africa in the hopes of securing slaves to work his newly found plantation in "Brasil."

It's easy to look back at writers like Defoe and be horrified (or even laugh at the absurdity) of the way in which they write about race. It's important to view these work within their appropriate historical context, although it should be noted that writers from the mid-seventeenth century that predated Defoe like Aphra Behn had spoken out against slavery. But it's not enough to recognize the inherent racism of *Robinson Crusoe* and move on. Later in the book Crusoe enslaves Friday, a native of the region, and while within the lens of history we see how such a narrative moment could logically come from the pen of Defoe, it's important to turn that spyglass around and look back the other way at where we are now because of foundational stories like these that still reverberate today.

Robinson Crusoe's beliefs about nature extend to his beliefs about other races—indeed, other races are seen as part of nature. By making nature the submissive subject of his desires, Robinson Crusoe establishes the classic paradigm of racist ideology that fueled slavery, the genocide of Native Americans at the hands of early settlers, and even debates today about black welfare moms and young African American men in prison as well as informed the western, expansionist view of nature as a thing to be exploited. Because the land was wild, uncultivated, and not brought to industrious purpose, it is *purposeless*, according to Robinson Crusoe—a thing to be feared, controlled, and ultimately owned.

The same goes for the "savage" races—to the eye of the European and American, their lifestyles and cultures had no apparent value or importance, and therefore to be made useful they must be subjugated and controlled for greater purpose. Usually the reason given was to bring them into the light of Christianity, but that argument was just a smokescreen for the more practical, worldly aims of colonized economic gain.

BOOKSMARTS

The great environmental debate of the past hundred years and the great race debate are not separate issues. We can find one single seminal germ of them both in *Robinson Crusoe*.

I should note here that, as previously stated, despite its racist nature, I really enjoyed much of *Robinson Crusoe*. I also like Rudyard Kipling, despite some pretty unsavory remarks he's made about other races being "half devil, half child." These authors are products of their time and should be judged accordingly. But there's no doubt that stories like *Robinson Crusoe* are foundational in our literature, thus they inform our very culture.

In the past few years we've had a spate of films—*Cast Away, All Is Lost, Life of Pi,* and even *In the Heart of the Sea*—that deal expressly with this basic tenet: a person, alone, at odds with nature, provides the narrative tension, which is released only once nature has been overcome and civilization regained. Understanding the way in which nature is comprehended and presented in these stories is vital to interpreting our culture, and how we talk about them and which stories we choose to teach is one of the most important choices we can make as educators and parents.

What are we actually teaching when we teach kids literature? Plot, mechanics, narrative, story, a bit of history maybe. But we all understand there's also a moral component. Books are suggestive blueprints for how to act, or at least helpful calculatory algorithms to use in plotting our course through life. There's been quite a bit of robust argument over this hypothesis. I personally fall on the side of John Gardner, who in the book-length essay *On Moral Fiction* argues that exploring some universal morality is the highest purpose of art.

There are teachers I've met who do an outstanding job teaching about race. But reading Baldwin's essays in *Notes of a Native Son, The Absolutely True Diary of a Part Time Indian* by Sherman Alexie, *Things Fall Apart* by Chinua Achebe, or *Invisible Man* by Ralph Ellison allows readers to absorb the story in such a way that it becomes part of their own identity. It's combined with the very DNA of their imaginations and gives rise to a new subspecies of ideas.

The same is true for books about nature and the wilderness. If we can see books—and the complex, imaginative projection that students engage in when they read or listen to stories and imagine they are within the fictional world, having the very same adventures—as an essential part of education, then we can use these books about nature to help our students' understanding of the environment, and perhaps more importantly their connection to it.

Other books—such as *Julie of the Wolves* or *My Side of the Mountain*, both by Jean Craighead George—tell a different story of nature. Students reading these stories may want to propel themselves into nature—as the heroes of both those stories do—and experience, even if only in pretend, imaginative play, the stories the novels represent. Coupling these books with long stretches of time in the outdoors, without some agenda, gives them the opportunity to figure these books out themselves. It allows the students the space, and time, and gives them the agency to come to terms with ideas of selfhood and nature and struggle on their own terms.

But if we don't give them that time—if we don't let go and allow them large chunks of their education to be spent outdoors—then they don't get to rework the very books they've read into their own imaginative DNA. They don't get to see that novels and stories are the most acute and far-reaching tools for discovering self. They see them as assignments. One of the best ways to give them the time—one of the tools—is unmitigated time outdoors, something the Norwegians in particular have developed into something that bridge ideology and lifestyle.

"OPEN AIR LIFE"

Friluftsliv is a Scandinavian philosophy—and already we're on shaky ground, because friluftsliv more akin to a lifestyle than anything intellectual or epistemological—which posits that the most innervating life is that which is lived in the outdoors. Literally translated, friluftsliv means "open air life."

Let's specify a bit more. Friluftsliv is not necessarily climbing K2—though it could be, under certain circumstances. Friluftsliv is entering nature in the most simple, uncomplicated way possible. A Himalayan expedition is anything but uncomplicated, but there could easily be moments of friluftsliv on such a trip: watching the morning sunrise, staring idly at a glacier, wandering among scree fields. But the concept of friluftsliv is inherently agenda-less—it has a surprising dash of Zen sensibility to it. The point is just to get outside and be outside, surrounded by nature, and be mindful of the fact that you're there. Any grand schemes or chest-thumping quests are outside the bounds of friluftsliv. Understanding the philosophical importance of friluftsliv provides an essential ideological underpinning for allowing students large tracts of time spent exploring outdoors.

The best example is a toddler in the woods. A toddler unconsciously exhibits all the central tenets of friluftsliv, wandering around exploring and being in the moment. It is the wellspring from which radical philosophies such as Arne Naess' deep ecology, Rachel Carson's ethos, and Bill McKibben's brilliant and trenchant environmental screeds have their beginning. Understanding it as a concept to be enacted rather than dissected is essential to unraveling its meaning.

As a philosophy it was a way for Swedes and Norwegians to actualize the concepts of nature heralded in Romantic poetry. Industrialization gave birth to leisure time, and a movement associated loosely with an outdoorsy cultural identity was born. As the nineteenth century became the twentieth, the concept was used to promote commercial tourism. The newest iteration of the concept within Scandinavia is anti-tourist, however, and is used to foster authentic experiences in nature rather than superficial "visits."

The first time the word was used in print is in Henrik Ibsen's poem "On the Heights." Ibsen, a Norwegian, wrote the poem sometime around 1859—just a year after he was married.

> In the lonely mountain farm,
> My abundant catch I take.
> There is a hearth, and table,
> And friluftsliv for my thoughts.

Ibsen's "On the Heights" is about a young man who leaves his mother and bride behind for the heights of the mountains, and watches the valley below as their homes burn to the ground. It is a tragic lyrical ballad, almost epic in length (387 lines) and in subject matter deals with a theme and subject matter that is prevalent in much of Ibsen's work: the artistic individual, fighting against the strictures of society, with freedom as the ultimate ideal. This freedom is personified by friluftsliv.

The second appearance of the word in print occurs in Ibsen's play, *Love's Comedy*. It is the story of love between Svanhild and Falk. Svanhild has chosen a marriage of convenience with a suitor, and Falk, a poet and teacher, is left grappling with the loss of his true love. Toward the end of the play, Svanhild leaves behind the possibility of being with Falk:

> SVANHILD looks after him for a brief moment, and says quietly but firmly:
> Now I shall put aside my friluftsliv; The leaf is falling; let the world receive me!

By putting aside her friluftsliv, Svanhild has given up independence, identity, and agency. Through its birth with Ibsen, friluftsliv came to represent a freedom of mind, actions, and individuality. This was especially important as Europe, and America, hurtled headlong into the industrial age, where the role of the individual in consumer-oriented, industrial society was being examined by writers like Marx. It was also a resistance to the worldview that Descartes had initiated hundreds of years prior; that nature was in fact a tool of man to be controlled.

Nowhere do we find the American equivalents of friluftsliv more than in the writing of Henry David Thoreau and John Muir; both writers central to American environmental thought, and the educational corollary of environmental education. In fact, even though friluftsliv is essentially a Norwegian concept, its literary standard bearers and contemporaneous advocates were Muir and Thoreau, who began espousing the ideals of friluftsliv at the same time the word grew in meaning in Scandinavia, though they never used the term. There is a dramatic connection between those two writers and philosophical ideas of friluftsliv, and it's no coincidence—it's evidence of a cultural and literary shift that occurred in the mid-nineteenth century that was radical, anti-authoritarian, and egalitarian to the extreme. This shift embraced nature as it is, rather than as it could be or should be. It was also grounded in social activism—Muir's aid in creating public parks like Yosemite provided access to the natural world for everyone.

Muir wrote about friluftsliv in books like *My First Summer in the Sierra* and *The Mountains of California*. In *The Mountains of California*, Muir writes about the purity of nature in a way that resonates with the philosophy of friluftsliv:

Climb the mountains and get their good tidings. Nature's peace will flow into you as sunshine flows into trees. The winds will blow their own freshness into you, and the storms their energy, while cares will drop away from you like the leaves of Autumn.

Thoreau too, especially in *Walden*, wrote of the positive effect of being in nature, and of the mindset required to experience it. "We need the tonic of wildness . . . At the same time that we are earnest to explore and learn all things, we require that all things be mysterious and unexplorable, that land and sea be indefinitely wild, unsurveyed and unfathomed by us because unfathomable. We can never have enough of nature." In fact, the subtitle of *Walden*, "A Life in the Woods," is a serviceable definition of friluftsliv.

The mid-1800s brought about a fundamental shift in how people viewed themselves in relation to nature, and this was exactly the same period that many of the underlying conceptual structures of modern education took root as well. In one sense, the very nature of humanity—what constituted a human being—was called into question as the rise of institutionalized, mechanized production and industry created workers who functioned only as part of the production process. Many nineteenth-century authors explored this. H. G. Wells' *Time Machine* imagined a future where workers became subhuman—the ape-like Morlocks—and live in a subterranean world running the machinery of production that supports the docile, weak Eloi (descendants of the upper class). Shelley's *Frankenstein* also explores these changing definitions, and challenged the idea of just where humanity, life, death, and science interact. Friluftsliv counteracted this notion of human-as-cog, and repatriated humanity back to the wilderness from whence we came.

Muir wrote: "When we try to pick out anything by itself, we find it hitched to everything else in the Universe." Friluftsliv shines a light on the interconnectedness of things. The fractal nature of the wilderness aesthetic encourages thought in a metaphoric way. For instance, the way the line of waves on the beach is reproduced in the undulating line where the vegetation meets the sand, as well as the topography of the coastal mountains. All the same pattern, fractally represented.

In our modular, post-modern, indoor world, these connections are hard to see, harder still to write about. In her Pulitzer Prize–winning book, *A Pilgrim at Tinker Creek*, Annie Dillard said she wanted to "write about the world" before she got tired of it. That book, and so many others, owe their existence to the tradition of friluftsliv and its progenitors Muir and Thoreau, and to the idea of noticing nature.

For some—one thinks here particularly of Muir and Thoreau—interiority is most acutely activated by experiencing the outdoors or wilderness. Only through prolonged exposure to the wild does interiority become uniquely accessible. It is not merely what we think about, but where we are when we do. Inward interiority is often seen as separate from the environment—but for adherents of friluftsliv environment and interiority are inextricably linked.

THE NATURE OF BOOKS

The eagerness evinced in nineteenth-century literature to get back to a rapidly disappearing natural world had its aesthetic counterparts. Because the reductionism of Cartesian philosophy had ruled for so long—and that scientific thought was believed to be able to "tame" and explain everything wild—there was a vacuum for art that celebrated and elevated natural, untrammeled places. Painters like the Luminists and Hudson River School in the United States began painting idyllic scenes of a rapidly disappearing natural world—that celebrated wild (though highly idealized) wilderness settings.

Humanity had spent such a long time trying to civilize itself that it lost sight of the essential truth that Muir and Thoreau wrote about—that we act in concert, in conspiracy, with nature and the wild—not against or apart from it.

Muir and Thoreau, as well as the protagonist of Ibsen's "On the Heights," are interesting in that they must work against the dominant paradigm of the nineteenth century: work is good, almost God. No century buzzes with activity and production quite like the nineteenth. In my own state of Vermont, the 1800s transformed a forested wilderness into a place overrun with sheep where over 90 percent of the state was pasture, textile mills crowded the rivers, and the trade routes to Boston, Montreal, Albany, and New York were full of goods being produced and shipped, hauled, and loaded.

Friluftsliv for Muir and Thoreau meant that they had to swim against the current of the day. They were seen by many as cranks and eccentrics. This is equally true today, where those who commit themselves to an "open air life" can be seen as aberrant or strange. While there is a nascent movement afoot—the popular book *Last Child in the Woods* by Richard Louv coined the term "nature deficit disorder"—the philosophy of friluftsliv is up against some serious competition in the form or smartphones, tablets, and laptops. In our world of multitasking and downloading and hi-speed Wi-Fi access, there is no app for friluftsliv, and it remains one of the clearest expressions of something central to our concept of humanity: freedom.

During the Romantic period, the relationship writers had with the earth was at once a totally distant, academic understanding and a vital reworking of the view of how humans interacted with their natural environments. Often nature was seen as an almost biblical Eden, or the very real struggles and difficulties that came from living in harmony with nature were overlooked. In the book *Dust,* which reviews western culture's appreciation and abhorrence of grit, dirt, and grime, the author writes: "Nineteenth-century Romantics, preferring the earthy people to the middle class, equated dirt with all things basic. Dirt—as soil, earth, and even manure—was for them the lands substance and the nation's moral nutrient."

How much does literature have to tell us about our relationship to nature—and what impact does that have on how we experience the wild with students? There can be little doubt that literature—novels, plays, stories, and poems—comprises an integral part of our collective cultural understanding. The tropes, themes, ideas, and philosophies espoused in literature inform the way we think about ourselves, the world, each other, learning, and teaching. Books have a great deal to tell us about how we view nature—how we *teach* nature.

Kurtz's Classroom

Joseph Conrad's *Heart of Darkness* speaks volumes about how to view nature—its corrupting influence, its irrationality, its madness. At once a volley aimed at the injustices of colonialism and a reaffirmation of racist ideologies, *Heart of Darkness* is a complex platform upon which a complicated view of nature is upheld. Its antecedents such as the film *Apocalypse Now* are central to the way our collective consciousness grapples with the natural world, its secrets, and influences.

The story of *Heart of Darkness* unfolds on a small boat at anchor in England. The crew is waiting for a shift in the tide, and one of them, a man named Marlow, begins to tell a tale of the horrors he witnessed in the Belgian Congo as a steamer captain on that country's eponymous river. Marlow tells the story of steaming upstream to the very last outpost of the Europeans, a station that operated under a man named Kurtz. Kurtz is depicted as a godlike figure throughout, a man capable of controlling the various tribes of the region and collecting more ivory—the raison d'etre of the colonial occupation—than any other agent on the river.

Conrad's writing is pretty dense as well as being beautifully evocative and philosophically compelling. As Marlow tells his tale of his journey up the river deeper and deeper into the jungly wilderness of the Belgian Congo, readers are drawn along in his wake. The sense of a deepening, eerie gloom persists as the steamboat makes its way upriver; the heavy sense of a shroud being laid over the boat advances until the steamboat is literally locked in my fog, a mysterious mist, by the time they're steamed to within a few miles of the enigmatic Kurtz's station deep in the wilderness. Conrad's description of nature veers from the sort of landscape description that accompanies much nature writing to something much more ominous:

> Going up that river was like traveling back to the earliest beginnings of the world, when vegetation rioted on the earth and the big trees were kings. An empty stream, a great silence, an impenetrable forest. The air was warm, thick, heavy, and sluggish. There was no joy in the brilliance of the sunshine. The long stretches of the waterway ran on deserted into the gloom of overshadowed distances. On silvery sandbanks hippos and alligators sunned themselves side by side. . . . And this stillness of life did not in the least resemble a peace. It was the stillness of an implacable farce brooding over an inscrutable intention. It looked at you with a vengeful aspect.

The tension builds as the steamer slowly and leakily chugs its way upstream to Kurtz's station. Marlow and his shipmates—some are natives he calls "cannibals," others whites he refers to as "pilgrims"—come under attack at one point by local natives. But finally they make it to the deepest, most remote part of the territory, and we meet the inscrutable Kurtz in all his weirdness.

How to describe a character like Kurtz? What a brilliant creation. Marlon Brando does the persona justice in *Apocalypse Now*. Kurtz is sick, we find, and as Marlow speaks with the only other European on that stretch of the river—a man who reveres Kurtz like a god—we learn that Kurtz is a brilliant but troubled man, and readers get the sense that Kurtz has performed gruesome deeds, possibly held sacrifices, and engaged in all manner of nasty, uncivilized behavior. Marlow tries not to fall under the sway of Kurtz, but even he finds himself taken aback in awe in meeting him. Kurtz seems to embody the greed of European imperialism, but is also described as being corrupted by nature—imbuing a kind of evil that Conrad suggests is lurking in the heart of the forest:

> The wilderness had parted him on the head, and, behold, it was like a ball—an ivory ball; it had caressed him, and—lo!—he had withered; it had taken him, loved him, embraced him, got into his veins, consumed his flesh, and sealed his soul to its own by the inconceivable ceremonies of some devilish initiation.

Sounds like a fun camping trip. Reading Conrad, it seems clear that when a human is left to confront nature, it drives them mad.

Of course, one of the great ironies in Conrad's view of nature is that he represents Kurtz as alone and at odds with it. Nothing could be further from the truth; the jungle along the river to the station is bursting with natives, peopled and full of human beings. This is the core racist ideology of Conrad's work. Kurtz is cut off from all *rational* and *civilized* life, thus it drives him mad.

This isn't to say that Conrad—given the age in which he was writing (*Heart of Darkness* was first published in serial form in 1899, and was based on real experiences Conrad had had on the Congo River)—didn't also deliver a serious criticism of imperialism and colonial racism. He does, but inherent in his descriptions is the brutality and corrupting influence of the wilderness, and he equates the local Congolese tribes with that wilderness, makes them a part of it, thereby condemning them to its evil.

It's both fair and unfair to levy this criticism against Conrad for his racist portrayal of black Africans. The fact is Conrad was hypercritical of the exploitive actions taken by colonial powers, but also a man of his time. However, Montaigne, the first essayist, was writing in the sixteenth century in a much more nuanced way about "cannibals" than even Conrad, despite the fact that Montaigne lived in a time in which views about other races was even more imbedded in racist thinking. In his essay "On Cannibals," Montaigne writes of "savages" thus:

> They are savages in the same way that we say fruits are wild, which nature produces of herself and by her ordinary course; whereas, in truth, we ought rather to call those wild whose natures we have changed by our artifice and diverted from the common order.

Those changed natures are evident in Kurtz. Kurtz is more than just a man twisted by the darkness of the wilderness. He stands in for European exceptionalism and imperialism as a whole. Marlow expounds on Kurtz's self-deification in one particular passage:

> "My Intended, my ivory, my station, my river, my—"everything belonged to him. It made me hold my breath in expectation of hearing the wilderness

burst into a prodigious peal of laughter that would shake the fixed stars in their
places . . . the thing was to know what he belonged to, how many powers of
darkness claimed him for their own.

The darkness is human greed, hubris, violence, and yet as one journeys
upriver one gets more and more inculcated with the idea that in a state of
nature, isolated in the wilderness, there is something horrific in us that claws
its way out. That civilization is the only way to avoid the basest parts of our
beings. For Kurtz, it is too late. He's spent too much time in the deepest,
darkest part of the jungle, and he's infected with its madness. He is seduced
by the "mute spell of the wilderness" that spurs his "brutal instincts" and
"monstrous passions."

And yet through Marlow's tale, we see Kurtz as a European—schooled and
civilized—sickened and polluted by the very wilderness he sought to subdue. On his deathbed, as Marlow brings him aboard and the steamboat turns
around to chug back downstream, Kurtz delivers his final edict. He defines
a European and American sense of expansionism and progress that will be
drawn upon for decades—a shared cultural understanding that weaves its way
through the way we teach, learn, and think about nature and the wild. It's a
philosophy that leads to the slaughter, involuntary schooling, and exploitation
of indigenous communities, as well as the destruction of the environment in
the name of resource extraction. Conrad gives Kurtz the final word:

"'Oh, but I will wring your heart yet!' he cried at the invisible wilderness."

When novels like *Heart of Darkness* are taught in schools—and Conrad's
excellent book is a standard text for many upper-level high school English
classes—they are often used to elucidate history or tease out various strands
of inquiry such as racism, colonialism, and other sociopolitical values. The
way nature is represented is an equally rich vein to explore. For a high school
student that spends a great deal inside, playing video games, connected to
technology, the view of nature presented by Conrad can seem grim indeed.
Using the novel to draw parallels between the racist ideologies of colonialism and the environmental degradation of industrial expansion is a profound
way to get students thinking about the way in which nature is viewed through
such a complicated lens throughout western history: as an Eden; a place of
escape; an untamed land of savagery; even the very home of evil itself. But by
reading about the wilderness the reader also incorporates wildness into themselves; when we read we engage in sustained imaginative projection. When
I read *Heart of Darkness*, I'm right there next to Marlow, nudging the rusted-
out tub of a steamship upstream. Sometimes I am Marlow, inseparable from
his thoughts and fears. But readers also can be imbued with an understanding
of the forest around him, be it malevolent or not, and in doing so develop a
deep understanding—and, one hopes compassion—for the world of nature.

Chapter 6

Outside the Inbox

When we talk about education—particularly at the elementary and high school levels—we're often referring directly to instruction. We think about the kids, the classrooms, the books, the devices, the policies, and the budgets. We think about the time it takes for kids to get through school, the work they have to do, and the experiences that they're having. The learning that they're doing. At the college level, at least, there's another conversation that is becoming more prevalent as the years tick by and the level of digital interface in our lives increases: the way teachers spend their time.

As in any profession, the level of competence varies among teachers; some are creative, hardworking individuals who seek to create meaningful experiences for their students, and some lack the fundamental skills, personality, and motivation to engender a sense of wonder and intellectual inquiry in their classrooms. By and large, however, according to a number of recent studies reported on in the *Washington Post*, teachers work hard (fifty-three hours a week on average) and are paid 17 percent less than comparably educated professionals in other fields.

Many teachers care deeply about what they do, and feel compelled—called, maybe—to do the very difficult work of taking two dozen kids and getting them through the day with a minimal amount of mayhem, and trying to teach them something in the bargain. In higher education, if blood pressure levels and loudly voiced, finger-wagging gesticulations during department meetings are any indication, professors are deeply invested in learning, teaching, and education.

Not only do they care about their students, but more and more teachers are talking about the constraints on their time that come from technology, the changing nature of the job description, and the continued emphasis on being many things to many people—teacher, counselor, mentor, and parent. The common argument against this line of thinking is that teachers are indulging in undue complaints, despite what many would believe to be an enviable schedule (summers off, done by 3 p.m. and lots of vacations). The research doesn't bear this out, however. According to statistics collected and analyzed by the Bill and Melinda Gates Foundation, teachers spend an average of ten to eleven hours a day planning lessons, worrying about their students, reading books and articles, and trying with all their might to maintain some level of sanity and grace in front of a room full of young people.

Twenty years ago, before the ubiquitous presence of the internet, class preparation and the job of teaching was markedly different on a daily, quotidian basis. Teachers generally spent the time before class prepping—getting the lesson ready, scribbling information on the blackboard, collecting the necessary materials the class would need. The time before the students arrived was valuable in that it was relatively undistracted; teachers had the opportunity for reflection, for calming, for some form of mindfulness.

Fast forward to present day. The daily dictates of the teaching profession have changed right along with the manner in which students have changed. Everyone is wired. Virtual lesson plans, emails from parents, colleagues, administrators—the value of quiet, contemplative time has been replaced with constant connectivity. This is true across educational levels.

The manner in which the computer (and email in particular) has changed the daily experience of the teacher cannot be underestimated. Among the many defects, the introduction of the internet and the way educational technology companies have monopolized teachers' time have diminished focused, intentional time spent on thinking about and planning for students, as well as reduced teacher's movement. Before, there may have been collegial discussion, trips to the library, or simply a quick stroll to loosen up before class; now, teachers are stationary, checking email.

When I get to the office, I often find myself switching on my computer and opening my email. I'm eager for that little dopamine rush when I open a particular message that bodes well, hungry for something novel or interesting. And then—shockingly quickly—I slide down into a clicking, archiving, catatonic state (it's ironic that when you save an email it's called "archiving," as though the messages I receive are these important artifacts rather than ads for erectile dysfunction and hair loss products). I end up wasting a bunch of time sorting through my inbox.

But it's more than that. My brain—muzzy with that pleasant, pre-caffeinated haze in which amorphous ideas dance with leftover wisps of last night's dreams—is intruded. My psychic space, which is much needed for the work that lays ahead of me, is invaded by all sorts of competing agendas and ideas. Without email, my brain is concerned with how to break down Montaigne's essays for students and get them to construct their own arguments as compellingly; or how to see in the structure of Jamaica Kincaid's *A Small Place* there is more going on than just really long sentences. Or perhaps I have a challenging student, one of the ones that is smart but is screwing up royally, and if I could just say a combination of the right things, I might deflect their trajectory of self-sabotage.

But now the interiority of my brain has visitors. Every email I click crowds the space between my ears even more. The assistant director of the library has asked me to fill out a Survey Monkey on library resources. The HR director is updating me about my benefits package. There's a message from the campus health center that someone in my 11:00 a.m. class has strep. The agenda for the division meeting is available for comment. I haven't met with my advisees yet, and the dean is waiting for an update. New Balance is having a sale on the shoes I really like. My colleague found an article on the *Huffington Post* I could totally use for class, if only I had time to read it and figure out what to do with it.

The answer to this conundrum is obvious: just don't check your email. I wish I was that strong. I'm not. I know some people have the self-control to limit their time clicking uselessly around their inbox. I am not one of them. I'm addict-like with email. I check it compulsively. I'm an impulsive person anyway, and if there's a laptop, with an email account attached to it, I find myself checking it all the time.

But there's another level in how teachers have to regulate their time in terms of email. Not responding promptly can make it appear like you're slacking. There could be an important request from the dean, the provost, the president! The culture we live in—especially in higher education—is coming more and more into line with the modern business, meaning that instant communication (and instant gratification) is the name of the game.

Regardless of what profession is examined, email has become the primary means of communication among people working together. Teaching is no exception. There are many reports and surveys trying to capture just how much time, exactly, professionals spend writing and reading email, but the average is a few hours a day—anywhere from two to five. This amount of time is sizeable regardless of the occupation or field. However, there are individuals who are resisting the domination of email as the primary vehicle for communication. Ironically, more often than not, they are actually part of the tech industry.

The other reality connected to the dominance of email and internet culture is that it necessitates large amounts of time spent indoors, sedentary. When time could be used before to get outdoors for a bit, walk around, perhaps even take a book and go sit under a tree to refresh the mind's understanding of a particular class text, now distraction and the imperative of constant connectivity keep teachers indoors. Teachers and student are equally denied the right to be outdoors by the incessant tug of the perception that email and work done in front of the screen hold more value than experiencing the quotidian adventure of the everyday outdoor world. Not everyone, however, has succumbed to the domination of the inbox. There are holdouts.

#NOEMAIL, NO BULLSHIT

Paul Jones looks like a wizard, writes erotic poetry, and helped invent the first electronic campus mail program. Despite the fact that he helped create one of the first electronic messaging programs used on campuses decades ago, Jones has one other interesting quirk: he doesn't use email anymore. He thinks it's stupid.

But Jones isn't some Appalachian hippie wearing home-woven flaxen knickers. A professor with a dual appointment at the University of North Carolina's School of Media and Journalism *and* the school of Information and Library Science, Jones is deeply engaged in digital technologies—just not email. He was co-chair of the 2010 World Wide Web conference, and claims to personally own a copy of the world's first web page. I messaged him on Facebook one morning about having a phone chat, and at first the only response I got was an emoticon of a sleepy-eyed smiley face yawning. "In line for coffee," he later wrote back.

When we finally spoke, Jones explained his "#noemail" campaign to me. Jones sees email as a time-waster and an ineffective way to communicate. While he is deeply interested in new forms of media, social networks, and digital learning resources, he sees email as a ridiculous tool to use, especially in a learning environment.

While we come at it from different angles—Jones is interested in the speed and efficiency of other forms of communication, whereas I want to be able to get outside more—it turns out that the net result for both of us is the same. We're not cloistered in an office.

"Email is designed for stationary workspaces," Jones explained to me. With the advent of mobile, even wearable, technology, the idea of having to be anywhere to do work seemed ancient to Jones. But Jones also represents an interesting paradox. Though he is immersed in the digital world, his reasons for not using email are actually closer to an analog rationale. He claims he's "more available to students," and that he has more time to reflect, to write, and to think. One of the things Jones kept bringing up was mobility. He spends more and more time walking around campus, having unplanned chats with students and colleagues. He simply moved around more, since he doesn't have to rush back to the office to check email. But he wasn't just walking, he claimed: "I think better walking than sitting."

One of the key components of the work Jones has engaged in over the past few decades is the way the world has shifted through technologies, and the way that has disrupted our own pre-digital lives. "I'm interested in the changes we bring to technology, and the changes technology brings to us," he said.

The interesting thing about removing email and replacing it with something non-digitally mediated is that it forces interaction and movement. If there is a message to deliver, the most available device pre-internet was the phone—where one could have an actual conversation where voice inflection, tone, and nuance can be used—or office memos were delivered, or even letters to various individuals throughout the workplace. In order to communicate, people had to engage in moving their body and opening up to experience.

How many novel, fortifying experiences are to be discovered walking from one office to another, from one part of campus to the next? From moment to moment, arguably not many, but if all the small interactions, the dozens of those moments a week, over a few decades of work, are combined, it's likely that reducing the amount of time spent in front of a screen increased the numbers of experiences to be had, and those experiences were with other people—talking, joking, arguing, and engaging. Workers could get outside more, and those few minutes of sun and light and air a couple times a day add up to a life spent in an environment that suits human beings and that is essential for our physiology and psychology. There is more actual life to be lived outdoors than in.

There is the potential that increased face-to-face interaction, exposure to the outdoors, and the experience of serendipitous moments have a positive effect on human cognition, including the development of empathy, increasing the hippocampus, and spurring positive neurochemical production of synapses. There is an argument to be made that movement, the outdoors, and human contact make better teachers. And this may be the key point.

The way that digital distraction removes teachers from both the way they want to teach, and the way nature can be used as a tool to develop students'—and *teachers'*—sense of self. By removing the interface of technology, teachers simply have more time to get outdoors, and the time they spend out there is more conducive to the sorts of interactions that fosters a real sense of learning; face-to-face chats, solitary rumination, or tactile engagement with the environment. Email takes time, but it also takes away time from being outdoors, which is anathema to learning.

MODELING ANALOG AWESOMENESS

The change in the educational lives of students starts with how teachers represent their own behavioral attitudes and cultural influences. How teachers model learning is vital—from kindergarten on through higher education. If the default mode is to stand at a wired-up podium, clicking through slides or showing videos, students will assume that learning follows the same format. But if teachers release themselves from Blum's "cage" and head out into the open, they are offering a very different blueprint to students on how to learn, explore, and discover the world, and themselves, anew.

At the core of this situation is a central tenet of teaching and being a teacher—the idea of modeling or being a mentor. This concept is notably different from just teaching information, and its relationship to the way that teachers spend their times bears on any discussion of the outdoors and its connection to learning.

Students view teachers through a variety of lenses. Sometimes, no doubt, teachers are seen as harbingers of doom. At other moments they may be viewed as something akin to family. It runs the gamut, but what seems clear is that *who* teachers are and *what* they do matters. How do teachers spend their time; do they walk the walk or only talk the talk? There's a long tradition of teachers existing outside the bounds of the commonplace. Some of the most compelling portraits of teachers in literature and film often depict someone who is at odds with the dominant paradigms of governance, the economy, or repressive social narratives. This is essential: teachers have long stood as an alternative to the pressures of conforming to the demands of society. There is always a balance between being part of the establishment and being apart from it, teaching in a way that eschews the dictates of pecuniary values or arbitrary decorum.

Within higher education this balance is still present. I have a colleague, Chuck, who goes about barefoot with wild, Einsteinian hair, gesticulating and shouting and making his students sit outdoors, in circles, shouting Latin mottos. He's brilliant, and one of the most deeply loved teachers I've ever known. Students respond to his refutation of the rules of decorum. This sense of radicalism is essential if we want students to buy into our particular pedagogies or message. This is not about political polarization, but rather a willingness to exist at the fringe of contemporary thinking and learning. The outdoors offers such an easily attainable forum for just this kind of experience—unstructured nature removes hierarchy and replaces it with authentic relationships. At the very center of this desire within our students to see teachers as "other" is their understanding that as children they are at odds with the adult world; seeing a teacher who also exists if not at odds, at least perpendicularly to the dominant hierarchies of the adult world is a way to engage them—to bring them to the table, so to speak, out of curiosity if nothing else.

Being outdoors—embracing it for all its basic values of health but also for its metaphorical importance as a place outside the bounds of adult control—is a powerful way to access this dynamic between child and adult, student and teacher. How compelling can a teacher be if the very experiences that make them who they are are reduced to the hypnotic interface experienced in front of a screen?

The usual argument is that the digital forum has so completely enmeshed itself into the modern world that to deny it—to not embrace technology as the primary means of teaching and learning and living—is to fall out of step with the times and to live in denial. Parts of this message are simply the boosterism of corporate software companies, filtered down through advertising and cultural identity, and part of it may be true.

If schools' job is to educate students, and the contingencies and requirements of daily life are moving more and more online, doesn't it stand to reason that they should embrace the digital medium both as teachers and individuals? In fact, many in education would disagree—at least partly. Because of humans' basic evolutionary background—a social primate who's evolved to respond primarily to social cues based on real, face-to-face relationships—people are wired genetically to respond to other humans. But more than that, despite Hollywood's efforts to make the hacker seem cool, and represent the geek at the keyboard as some kind of hero (which they may be), the fact remains that students respond to teachers most notably when they model autonomy, independence, and freedom.

The demands of digital distraction leave little room to represent this dualism. If teachers are constantly on iPads, if they are held in somnambulant sway by the swirl of corporate-produced digital tools and entertainment, and if, when students see their teachers, on a daily basis, hunched over a screen tapping away, teachers aren't seen as the sort of mentors, or leaders, that inspire learning. They're seen as complicit.

The final connection here between taking the measure of teachers and the role of narrative in learning is key. Stories are, arguably, one of the most powerful vessels of learning. A narrative like *Robinson Crusoe* or the story of Frederick Douglass offers such rich territory to cover from an educational perspective. I've never met a student yet who doesn't love a good tale. We are narrative creatures for whom the arc of a good story is as familiar as the curve of our own instep. But not only can stories from books compel a deeper understanding in students, reflecting on their own stories and experiences is a highly valuable learning tool as well.

My stories come from the outdoors. I've never told a very good story about something I've done online. I'm always a little bored when someone begins to tell me about some digital escapade. They posted this and someone commented with that and the battle of digital wits raged on. The media is full of articles about "Twitter feuds" that strike the reader as vacuous and vaguely depressing: is this what discourse has amounted to? I just don't find it very compelling. I don't think most of us do. When four African American students sat down at a Woolworth's lunch counter in Greensboro, North Carolina, and risked body and soul to push for desegregation, they created a dialogue that reverberates even today. A scorching rebuttal on Twitter? Who cares.

But I have noticed that when our students are given experiences in the wide-open world—and when we, as teachers, come back from the outdoors with stories—kids listen. They gravitate to us, eager to hear about *actual* things that happened. Travel books and adventure stories still stock the shelves at the bookstore—memoirs like *Eat, Pray, Love* and *Wild* are massively popular books about women who sought to have experiences out in the world, not slack-jawed in front of a screen.

Children yearn for the real like they yearn for a good story. Being outdoors gives us these stories. Being outdoors, ourselves, as teachers, gives us the tools to be better. Not just teachers benefit from the ability to become a raconteur of the wilds, but as parents, we come to occupy a space in our children's imagination quite different from the one when they come home and we're typing away at our laptops, monosyllabically pointing them in the direction of some microwaved snacks (guilty as charged). If parents—who, in reality, bear more of the weight of shaping children's attitudes and mores than even teachers—are to place themselves in a position of influence, rather than arbitrary authority, in the lives of their children, it is worthwhile to ask what sort of role the outdoors plays for parents in developing experiences for children, and how the encroaching omniscience of the internet is detrimental to exactly those types of foundational experiences.

THE INCORRIGIBLE REALITIES OF PROCREATION

Parenting—it's difficulties, humiliations, tedium, and time-usurping demands—came as a shock to me. I always knew I wanted to be a parent, and so all the good things such as snuggling on the couch reading together with my kids, bike rides to school, inventing weird cookie recipes, and wrestling in the grass came as no surprise. They were expected and loved. But in general, there have been moments of transcendent joy levied with agonizing stretches of repetition, boredom, mild irritation, visceral rage, and a barely suppressed selfishness on my part that I'm deeply ashamed of. In short, my experience as a parent is probably pretty similar to most people: peaks of awesomeness surrounded by valleys of crap.

I've made a decent effort to get my kids outdoors. Currently, I live in a place where that's easy to do. Vermont has a small-scale, accessible, open landscape with plenty of forests and lakes and mountains for play. But even when I lived in Los Angeles, my wife and I tried to get Vivien out to the beach, camping in Joshua Tree, or at least to the park for the afternoon. Going outside as a family has been our default activity. It's more or less free, doesn't require too much planning, and nobody seems psychologically scarred by the experience afterward.

But there is a growing threat in the form of digital screen–based entertainment that is already overwhelming families. More and more, children seek entertainment at all developmental levels through smartphones, iPads, and laptops. When children play, inevitably they end up in some basement room, playing Wii or watching movies. There is nothing particularly new about this experience. Television has long been the "electronic babysitter." But the way in which digital experiences are so pervasive now does represent a new paradigm; there is just *so much* screen-based entertainment available and so much is finely tweaked for rapid consumption that parents are faced with a whole host of digital distractions to contend with.

The common line of argument—from parents who have embraced these technologies as simply the "way things are" and particularly those who themselves are deeply wired—is that to lament some bygone day when children played outside is like crying over the fact dinosaurs no longer exist; it's a fait accompli, so get over it. Often, those who reject or question the dominance of the internet and screens as the default mode of entertainment and engagement get labeled as technophobes and an alarmist. But it is exactly that dismissive, condescending air with which people meet criticisms of the internet that is part of a deeply held cultural bias.

In his pervasively brilliant treatise on the subject, *The End of Absence*, Canadian author Michael Harris writes, "Interrogate the dominance of a mounting technopoly with anything more aggressive than cocktail conversation and you will swiftly be accused of 'moral panic'—which is one of those tidy terms that carries around its own moral imperative. One *must not panic*." The reality is many individuals are scared of technology and do feel a swelling anxiety very close to alarm.

IMAGINING LANDSCAPES

Children need to enter a fantastical world of their own to demark their lives from the staid predictability of the adult world. In order to do this, they need a literal landscape to explore. The very tactile, physical realness of the barren lot or backyard hedge is the ancillary soil of imagination—where it takes root and grows.

In the mind of a child, they *own* the woods and fields around their home—the topography of their imaginations and games is overlaid by the actual contours of the world around them. The borders and territories of childhood are as clearly delineated in their mind as the legal boundaries that reside in some drawer in the county clerk's office, but the borders and boundaries, features and transects are dictated by imaginary play, pretend worlds, and narrative. A bush with an empty, hidden interior becomes a fort, high tree limbs look-outs, muddy ditches jungle swamps.

When children play in the woods, and an adult comes tromping through, their very presence in the woods is an aberration. Their trespassing is not just physical. They invade the psychic space children create under drooping boughs of spruce and in thickets of crab apple trees, spoiling the tenuous balance of imagined worlds with their adult interference. The woods belong to children in a way that they'll never belong to adults—ownership without possession, the way that animals "own" the forest.

For children, the forests, or any unstructured, natural spaces, are places where games and imagination hold sway, not schedules and rules. The unmediated stretches of time children spend outdoors playing on their own represent the all too fragile vicissitudes of freedom and personal sovereignty—the brief ruling of a little kingdom of sumac and goldenrod.

Here, then, is where the outdoors comes into play and becomes not just some mildly healthful and beneficial activity for kids but a radical rejection of screen-based culture because ethernet cables will not stretch into the bramble and thicket between neighborhoods. Eventually, when children head out into the wild world, the devices become less and less important, and kids will find themselves outside the influence of digital distraction, beyond the reach of companies and commercial coercion. They'll be free, and roughly defining their minutes according to the world around and within them, thus, learning and thinking and experiencing the world and themselves in it. No screen can deliver that.

EN PLEIN AIR

In searching for the antithesis of this indoor, screen-focused life of learning, it's helpful to think about how the very idea of solitary reading, creativity, or thinking was viewed in the not-too-distant past to provide some grist for the mill. Despite the way that the internet makes it seem that everything is new under the sun (the internet functions both as a means for us to recall what we've forgotten and to entice us to something new), western art has experienced a similar moment in the past that can help us illustrate why a refusal to be confined indoors as teachers and educators may have a solid cultural precedent.

During the nineteenth century, artists, particularly painters, began to feel confined by the strictures of the European classical school of thought about "how you should paint." Similarly to the way that modern education has students and teachers stuck inside "teaching" and "learning" by pecking away at the keys on computers, with the whole experience modulated and dictated by educational software, artists of the nineteenth century had been told by the dominant institutions of the time that real art happened only in the studio. Real art came from strict instruction and adherence to the traditions of the academy. Within this oppressive environment there was little room for freedom, experimentation, and truth, so, artists being artists, many simply folded up their canvases and walked out the door.

It was in the midst of the grimy, smoke-filled, coal-fired nineteenth century that the artistic movement known as en plein air took flight. The French term simply refers to painting outdoors, in natural light. The Hudson River school of American painters embraced it, as did many impressionists. Artists like Renoir, Monet, Decamp, Ferenezy—they all departed from the confines of their studios to experience painting in the natural world, with the sun casting its glow over the earth. It was during this heady time when Impressionism redefined the world of art and photography began to make artists question what, exactly, the role of a portrait or landscape painter was that the en plein air phenomena picked up speed.

It was also at this time that artists began to paint what they actually saw. They began to go out, into the open air, and paint the world around them. And interestingly, what they often painted was women reading books outdoors.

There are two significant aspects of this tradition of painting women quietly flipping the pages of some book with their legs tucked up underneath them on a blanket beneath a willow tree or seated on a park bench.

The first is that while there are any number of paintings during the period that reflect this interest in the restful, female, outdoor reader, there is nothing that is particularly significant in terms of the symbolism, message, or cultural import of these moments. Unlike the way in which impressionists released themselves from the oppressive bonds of painting in a photorealist fashion, and simply chose to try and capture the essence of light, movement, and let their brush strokes be seen as a part of the painting, this collective group of women reading outdoors was a by-product of the work, rather than the focus. The impressionists in particular were simply heading out, easel over the shoulder, and finding stuff to paint, or asking long-suffering wives, sisters, and mothers to cop a squat and reread that old novel so they could sit still while they were painted.

The second—not particularly related to the artistic moment—is that the paintings of this period do, in retrospect, remind us that prior to the widespread use of indoor gas and then electric lighting, the best place to read a book was in the full light of day. The best place to read—and this is still the case—is in the soft light of the outdoors.

One of my favorites is by American painter Theodore Robinson, whose life spanned the latter half of the nineteenth century. Admittedly, I may be biased, as Robinson was born in 1852 in Irasburg, Vermont—my home state—but the painting has merit despite my favor. It's of a woman seated next to a little pond, a boat pulled up the reedy bank behind her. She sits comfortably on the bank reading, and the bold, red strokes of Robinson carve her jacket out from the green of the waterside. The book she holds in her hands practically dissolves into the light of the pond, and the water beckons in choppy, glistening stokes. The thing I like the most about this painting is the angle of her head as she reads. Her head is bent toward the book, and there's a little bit of lift to her elbows, like she's just found a really good, stirring part of the novel and is deeply absorbed in the action.

The women in these paintings are reading everywhere: on the side of the road, in the woods, in boats, in trees, in fields and mountains. And every time I see a painting like this, I am reminded of a simple, glaring fact: going into the outdoors was unexceptional, and the very reason the impressionists painted outside was to try and paint what you could actually see. And what they saw was women reading. The very unremarkable-ness is what makes it so remarkable.

The artists of the en plein air movement weren't trying, necessarily, to destroy all artistic traditions as they had existed to that point, nor was it necessarily, at the time, seen as the dynamic shift in the way that we think about art and impressionism today. And yet, in hindsight, it's easy to see the courage it took to reject the dominance of the art schools and launch forth into the world. But at the time, one wonders if it was a matter of more personal, prickly personal preference.

I've known a few artists, and the best of them seem to share the characteristic of not being particularly jazzed at being told what to do. A rather independent lot, and here I think we can draw a connection between the desire for teachers to be released from the confines of digital necessity and the movement of artists outdoors in the late nineteenth century to take in some light and air, a call for an en plein air education movement.

The move to take education—including the way teachers spend their time—outdoors more isn't part of some large-scale, revolutionary paradigm shift, but rather the practical emergence of a rational reaction to confinement. This is an important distinction, because while the argument that the desire to engage in education en plein air could be seen as some metaphysical exercise, it's not that, necessarily. It's just a pain in the ass to be stuck inside all day.

WILD AMERICA

For some, the wilderness doesn't necessarily inspire or provide some psychological or metaphysical lift. For many people the wilderness may not be particularly transcendent. Not everyone is required to go outside to access some form of ecstasy like John Muir, who flung himself about the Sierra in an orgiastic whirl of spiritual bliss. For many, time spent outdoors does not have that level of spiritual awakening. However, using the outdoors as means of providing balance is vital, as it can provide a sense of opposition and perspective.

Teachers, parents, and children can use the wild not to escape, or become someone else, but rather to become more fully themselves. It is possible to connect with some basic version of personhood—some primary level of self—when out in the world, brushing aside overhanging limbs and stepping over punky, rotten logs. While spending time outdoors may not provide some with a feeling of expansiveness and the sense that they're in flux and flow with some great organic harmony, there is the opportunity to become more calmly internalized and experience what essayist Sven Birkerts calls "that curling up into the self."

Only by entering the wild can we offer our children and students the experience of being *without*—against which to compare the bloating abundance in which the western world lives.

The materially focused, indoor life with all its parts—laptops, connectivity, the appearance of social acceptability—none of them will necessarily improve the ethical, intellectual, or personal development–related gains of our children. Neither are they benign. Particularly in the case of young children, the introduction of digital entertainment or "edutainment" can foster petty discrepancies of character, distracted anxiety, neurotic desire, and rev up the cycle of distraction that is plaguing students.

Every day in the modern world it has become the standard experience to rush chaotically about, checking email a dozen times, texting, and posting experiences to social media—curating a version of self that distracts us from the real thing (again, I'm not casting stones, but rather speaking anecdotally from experience). It seems as though this stretching of the self over multiple dimensions (real, digital, social) can reduce the solidity of our persona. The web can affect the sense of self—for children especially—as the One Ring affected Bilbo, making them feel "thin, sort of stretched, like butter scraped over too much bread."

Overusing the internet to demonstrate identity can diminish the child's sense of their own humanness, and their outright capacity to be *in* the world as an agent rather than *of* the world as an accomplice becomes more apparent.

The irony is that the more teachers engage in the digital interface of the internet, the more they appear to be engaged in the process of educating students. In fact, an online presence is deemed a requisite part of the job market—a necessary ingredient in a thinking person's life if they wish to be seen as active and engaged. In fact, the more there is acquiescence to digital culture, the more credibility is gained from students, colleagues, and peers.

It has become a requirement to demonstrate an understanding of digital communication, and imbue the self with the hip appeal of technology, evince being in-touch with the demanding narrative of the necessity of a digital infrastructure in the world. No longer is social capital based on experience and reflection, but rather technological aptitude is seen as the sine qua non of the life of a teacher.

For a brief time when I was a kid, I was a member of the local Boy Scout troop. I attended a total sum of one jamboree, somewhere in the neighboring Adirondacks. My memories of scouts are vague and hazy. I recall a clunky plastic Native American kerchief brooch-thing, worn and crudely painted. My scoutmaster was a soft, doughy middle-aged dad with Coke bottle glasses and wrangler jeans. We spent a lot of time sitting cross-legged on the floor in a circle, talking about how to follow a river downstream if we got lost in the woods. I didn't stick with it for very long, and my overall impression of the experience was that it was boring—sort of like school.

My interest in Scouts was hardly unique. The idea of the rustic, independent woodsman was a central component of the fantasies kids I grew up with engaged in. The fuel for these visions of adventure in the outdoor world were stories. Books were the primary tools used to navigate some sense of self. For much of twentieth-century history, children iconized the idea of the recently disappeared pioneer as an idealized version of themselves, fueled by books and television like *Little House on the Prairie*. A sort of rugged, American individualism pervaded the fantasies and cultural touchstones of children. It was not unusual for children, even as recently as the 1970s and 1980s, to aspire to some level of outdoorsy competence as a means of establishing an identity.

MOUNTAIN MEN AND PEDAGOGUES

The outdoors, and the characters imagined and imitated there, represented freedom and adventure and expansiveness, both of actual geographic terrain and of ideas. Indoors was the realm of adults, where things could get broken and rules had to be followed.

For many children growing up in the twentieth century, imagination was fueled by stories of the outdoors. Jack London's *White Fang* and *Call of the Wild*; Walter Farley's *The Black Stallion* and *My Side of the Mountain* by Jean Craighead George are all examples of the lure of the outdoor adventure. All of them took place outside, and had either animals or young kids as the heroes.

Books often catered to specific types of outdoor adventure; the child who loved stories of wolves and dogs could read a shelf full of stories such as canine-centric adventure stories of Jim Kjelgaard, whose books *Big Red*,

Snow Dog, and *Wild Trek* feed visions of an unrestrained, wild, adventurous life. These books often feature a hero, some strapping, outdoorsy woodsman who places a value on freedom and spurns the institutionalized demands of more civilized lives. There has been a long-standing national fascination with the unfettered woodsman and the unique freedom he (and it's usually a "he," unfortunately) represented.

On a certain level, the American identity was forged in conjunction with the exploration of the frontier during the eighteenth and nineteenth centuries. The iconic American character was often a woodsy, self-sufficient sort of person—an independent and resourceful individual who faced the challenges of the wild world with pluck and free-spirited vigor. Again, one thinks of Laura Ingalls Wilder's characters, especially the heroine of the *Little House* books and television show and of other iconic symbols of the American wilderness such as Davy Crockett and Daniel Boone.

In his deeply personal and penetratingly great collection of essays, *I Am Sorry to Think I Have Raised a Timid Son*, Kent Russell explores this notion of the "American Identity," but his particular focus is American masculinity. In fact, the title of his book is a quote attributable to the outdoor icon Daniel Boone himself, who wrote it upon disappointingly learning that his son did not sign up to fight in a battle as part of the local militia.

Russell's take on Boone is spot-on in terms of isolating two paradoxes that inhabit this notion of the outdoorsy, self-reliant person that so many kids who grew up in the twentieth century sought to emulate in some way. The first is that the premise of the "frontiersman," or "pioneer," is not just a caricature but rests on such a deeply flawed notion of history as to be criminal. For even cute little Laura Ingalls Wilder and her family were guilty of participating in a massive migration—the movement of colonial settlers from the New England coast to the west that brought about the genocide of Native Americans.

While there is a deep tradition of heroic stories of frontiersmen like Daniel Boone and Davy Crockett (who, according to the song, "kilt him a bar when he was only three"), for those growing up with these characters as models it was done without accepting the full weight of their legacy. It was people like Boone who trailblazed the wilderness for white settlers who would bring about the destruction of the Native Americans who already lived in said "wilderness." Plucky little Laura Ingalls Wilder's adventures were admirable and entertaining, but Pa had settled the family on land that was already spoken for. In other words, he stole it. Russell says it best when he writes, "Boone was a frontiersman, which is a latter-day euphemism for 'unrelenting opportunist.' He tramped around the native element looking for unclaimed resources, things to 'exploit before moving on.'"

Russell's descriptions of Boone sound exactly like the sort of characters that, for some, defined the very type of outdoor persona that encapsulated the relationship between outdoor adventure and freedom. The stories were replete with episodes kids in particular connected with: raising wolf pups, fighting bears, and surviving in the wild. As Russell writes, the legends surrounding these figures from the outdoorsy American imagination were "tall tales" indeed, fueling the drive for children to get outside and adopt the pose of the frontiersman, striding across the landscape "Boone could hold a long rifle in one hand and take the head off a nail from a distance. . . . Short and powerful, pony-built, he ran away from home after killing one of his father's horses in a jumping accident."

It is characters like this—Russell calls these violent, masculine icons "opaque brutes"—that many children (mostly male) idolized—either unconsciously or willfully ignorant of the fact that every story of pioneer bravery and adventure is a story of genocidal colonialism and the destruction of the Native American cultures that preceded it.

The second paradox that exists in this image of the roving woodsman is the inherent lack of self-reflection such a life, or person, would contain. In thinking about the legend of Daniel Boone as an actual person, Russell writes about the potential that Daniel Boone kept moving—shooting, hunting, trapping, scouting, and exploring—because he was afraid. "He feared that, were he ever to stop, the mind he needed to keep trained on a target might instead turn on him." This type of character, the ceaselessly venturing American ideal of the "woodsman," rests on this pivotal notion: that to be that person is to be without reflective capacity, without the sense of analysis that would bring the very adventures undertaken into clearer focus.

If these types were to stop and think, two things would happen. First, they'd have to reckon with the reality of killing animals for sport or food, and avoiding any moral judgment on that, there's still the very real and impossible to escape ethical argument they'd have with themselves about the right they may or may not have to snuff another being's life out like a candle. But more importantly, this sort of self-reflection was considered for many who bought into the American ideal of masculinity as a weakness. To be internally reflective was to be a softy—one of what Russell cynically calls "anemic ephebes." The paradox is that the last thing these characters were was "the kind who understands himself, explains himself, acquits himself" according to Russell.

This sort of self-reflective capacity and intellectualizing was given a name in the latter part of the twentieth century. Individuals who engaged in that sort of rumination were called nerds.

NERDS!

The question to be asked is what we've gained by embracing the culture idea of nerds or geeks—those who are socially a bit inept but deeply involved in the sort of critical inspection Daniel Boone would've scoffed at—and what we may have lost by losing the fantasy of the iconic woodsman. What has been discarded as America has moved away from the visions of outdoor adventure that once permeated the imaginations of children? Yes, they were flawed, but they were very much about connecting with the landscape and about exploring the outdoor world. Outdoor, imaginative play was physically and psychologically beneficial for children, and aided in emotional and social development. What is "nerdiness" good for and how has made an impact on outdoor play?

In a 2014 article from *The New York Times* titled "We're All Nerds Now," journalist Noam Cohen writes, "Never before has the boundary between geek culture and mainstream culture been so porous." Cohen goes on to cite numerous examples of the prevalence of geek, or nerd, culture and the way it's shifted conceptions of identity. The massive popularity of geek culture–based shows like "The Big Bang Theory" and the fact that most people are consumed by technology are evidence, according to the article, of a large shift in the perception of what was previously a marginalized culture. The fact is, with giants like Google, Apple, and Microsoft dictating much of our lives through technological interfaces, the age of the geek has dawned.

Much of what comes along with the rise of a culture that venerates geeky attributes like technical intelligence, specialized knowledge, science, and video games is positive. The age-old dynamic of the jocks beating up on the nerd with tape on his glasses has become stereotypical legend. Now the coolest pop culture symbols are often tech-savvy like the tattooed hacker in *The Girl with the Dragon Tattoo*.

The cultural reach has even infiltrated academia. A quick Google search of "nerd culture" brings about a veritable cascade of dissertations about geek culture and identity with titles like "Nerds: A Reclamation of an Identity," and "Why Be Normal? Language and identity practices in a community of nerd girls."

What is clear is that the age-old markers of childhood and adolescent "coolness" have changed. If my own anecdotal experience is at all telling, on the college campus I work at a programmer who spends sixteen hours coding is as likely to have social standing as the football quarterback. It's a radical shift. As a child, I admired and attempted to emulate heroes who moved through the world like Daniel Boone—who literally traversed the landscape—and had a worldly competence about nature and the creatures in it. Now, kids who can navigate the virtual worlds, create alternate versions of themselves through digital identities and avatars, and who are fluent in various online languages and social spheres are seen by their peer groups as mastering some new and exciting world.

And why wouldn't a kid take the technological route to forming an identity or navigating their social worlds? Tech thirty years ago was clunky or downright impossible to use unless you had an engineering degree. Now, with the user-friendly interface we find on smartphones and social media networks, kids have the option to upload Periscope videos and gain a following, post videos to YouTube and receive accolades, or interact with virtual peers online in gaming communities. And all this can be achieved with minimal real-world discomfort while sitting on the couch, mainlining Oreos and clicking and swiping their way into their newfound digital identities. None of the natural world's discomforts—bugs, physical effort, dirt, and the complicated, nuanced, and frustrating reality of playing or working in the unstructured natural world with others—need to be endured. *My Side of the Mountain* doesn't stand a chance against *The Matrix*.

NAKED NATURE

While children readily default to digital devices as a means of entertainment (my son is forever trying to discover my password to the laptop, watch television, and get my wife to film him throwing action figures and Barbies out the window in slow motion on her iPhone), the question remains whether it makes them *happier*. Clearly, the sedentary nature of most interaction with digital devices is unhealthy. But what about the psychological impacts? And beyond that, how is the imagination of our children being changed by the way that nature is more and more pixelated rather than experienced?

One of the most interesting facets of the rapidly evolving way the outdoor world has been incorporated into digital entertainments is the manner in which the understanding about the outdoors commonly held culturally is no longer based on personal experience, but rather through entertainment. This understanding (or lack thereof) filters down to schools and the way nature and the outdoors is approached pedagogically.

The television show *Naked and Afraid* has stripped down modern nature-based entertainment to its most elemental form. The Discovery Channel show is currently in its seventh season. The premise is simple: two "survival experts" are dropped somewhere in the wild to survive for twenty-one days. Each expert gets to bring one survival tool—fire starter or knife, usually—though sometimes one will bring an inexplicable item like a magnifying glass or parachute cord. One man, one woman, and they have to survive for the three weeks finding food, making shelters, and dealing with bugs, animals, and all the struggles of surviving in the wild. And they're naked.

It's a really interesting show. I admit here to being an avid watcher. It's totally absorbing melodrama—two personalities struggling in a difficult environment, with all the insecurities and personality traits on full display. No doubt what is watched at home on the television is a highly edited version of the truth, with manufactured narrative arcs and plenty of false theatrics aimed at boosting ratings. Regardless, it works, and is an intriguing show to watch.

Naked and Afraid digs into the modern psyche and taps into two great phobias—being naked in front of strangers and being lost in the wild. Both are deeply held cultural fears. Being naked (particularly in America, less so in Europe) is seen as a thing to be feared. The show probably wouldn't work in Germany or Scandinavia, where folks are less uptight about their dangly bits. And, of course, people are deeply afraid of the wilderness and the show does a great job with night vision, Blair-Witch-style nighttime dramas, with survivalists staring wide-eyed into the darkness as creatures (or their imaginations) go creeping and crashing through the woods.

Naked and Afraid owes much of its success to its thematic precursor, *Man vs Wild*, the Bear Grylls vehicle that has the British military personality eating grubs and surviving in some of the world's most iconic wildernesses: the Sahara, Amazon, and so forth. Between the two shows, hundreds of millions of viewers tune into the version of nature versus human. They represent a huge swath of the population, and the inherent structure speaks to a complicated relationship with nature and the way the western world filters its understanding of the wild. These shows, and others like it (*Survivor* comes to mind), bear on our conversations about how we as a culture view nature and how we teach it, and what the psychological impacts may be of that evolving perception of the wild world. (Remember, the Discovery Channel was originally an educational cable venture. In fact, there's an entire section of the corporation of the Discovery Channel called Discovery Education.)

Nature has become digitally fetishized through shows like *Naked and Afraid* and corporations like Discovery Education. Given that the boundary between TV and online entertainment has become vague to the point of inconsequence, it seems that the digitalization of nature has gained a solid hold on the American imagination. Whereas kids used to go play outside, they now watch an edited version of outdoor experiences in places they've never been. After watching Bear Grylls slide heroically down the sheer face of some spire-ridged Alaskan peak, or wade manfully through tea-colored jungle rivers, slapping aside crocs, what kid would want to explore that overgrown woodsy tract behind the drugstore? Better to passively absorb the wild through the screen then get out there and have to navigate the complications of the real world. The digital experience is just so much *easier*.

THE HABITAT OF CHILDREN

The brilliance of the internet lies in its rapacious, undiscerning appetite. It hoovers up everything: culture, ideas, concepts, trends, belief systems, ideologies, and fantasies, and digitally repackages them as two-dimensional entertainment. It flattens their affect, dilutes their impact, and impregnates them with corporate sponsorship. Turns everything fibrous to pap.

Real-life experiences, especially those in the natural world, give us insight into our characters in a way that virtual experiences just can't. We have bodies that are inextricably tied to the way we think and grow, feel and dream. If we allow education to follow suit, if we turn away from the classroom of nature and further embrace the digital forum as a means of interpreting the world, we run more than the risk of our students and children losing touch with the natural world; we run the risk of them losing touch with themselves.

There's an inverse relationship between spending more time outdoors with our children and students and the power of technology. It's so, so easy to go outside. Just open the door and go. And yet, it is so, so difficult to resist the lure of technology. We're neurologically hardwired to look for novel information, and fill knowledge gaps. In fact, one of the ways curiosity works as a motivating drive is to make us look for information when *we're not even sure what information we need or want*. If ever there was a description of the psychological state of clicking randomly around the internet, there it is.

The resulting tension can be exhausting. Teachers feel bound through administrative pressure and cultural expectations to wire the classroom. Parents find it easy (and get a much-needed break from their kids!) to just offer up digital distraction. And yet, what our culture loses by losing the intimate relationship children have with the outdoor world is precious: a sense of themselves as beings with agency, and the means to project themselves imaginatively into adventures that build their sense of self. Without those opportunities—without fighting to maintain them—what will our children remonstrate us for in decades to come? Possibly, it will be for not working harder to preserves the threatened habitat of childhood.

Chapter 7

Humanimal

The basic problem with civilization, development, progress, plastic lawn chairs, four-lane blacktop roads, and individual packets of microwaveable mac 'n cheese is that—despite their convenience—there's a consequence: the unintended smiting of Gaia.

The planet earth has had a hard time of it lately. Climate change, deforestation, massive pollution in its seas and underground; the brutal extraction of resources and the destruction of flora and fauna on an extinction-event level; the crowded, hungry clamoring of the human species, *Homo sapiens*, as people prod and poke every corner of the globe for more, more, more. We're like the neediest significant other ever. Earth should've dumped us a long time ago.

Despite this, the planet has been surprisingly resilient to human's overbearing greed. The fact that Amur tigers still stalk the land and creatures like orcas and krill and monarch butterflies still exist is nothing short of a miracle. Humans are seven billion strong and counting—rapacious, shortsighted, and mostly preoccupied with feeding the mouths around us, and hoping for a better tomorrow in the form of a new water well, better cooking implements, a radio, an iPad, or a souped-up Porsche. Extreme omnivores, we eat anything and everything. Brilliant builders, we've cleared the land to create monuments to our intellect and civilization like the Great Wall of China and the Taj Mahal, as well as symbols of our insipid hubris like Dubai's man-made Palm Island. We've learned to take the very stuff of the earth in the form of minerals and radioactive elements and create engines that have propelled us into space and down the Vegas Strip.

The question isn't how long the earth can support us; the question is how it is possible it's supported us thus far?

Before you think me some wild-eyed, delusional enviro-hippie alarmist, let's check out some grim statistics.

According to various sources such as magazines and organizations like *The Guardian*, National Geographic, CNN, and the National Science Foundation, the extinction rate—the number of species that are killed off, forever, each year—is somewhere around 0.01 percent and 0.1 percent. This sounds almost heartening. I mean, I wouldn't sweat a 0.01 percent increase in the interest rate of my mortgage. But it's actually rather terrifying when you consider just how many species that is.

A further glitch is that we don't actually know how many species our planet contains. Every year there seems to be a few articles about some intrepid team of post-docs who count the beetles on some tree in a god-forsaken jungle somewhere and discover that about 90 percent of the species are unknown to science. But, for the sake of argument, let's say there are two million different species of creepy-crawly on the planet, from nematodes to elephants. That means that between 200 and 2,000 species go extinct *every year*. Two hundred Amur tigers, 2,000 resplendent quetzals—gone forever. Whichever stat is right, that's a pretty scary number.

Species have always gone extinct as the planet changed, but the rate of change today is 1,000–10,000 the rate of what scientists refer to as the "background extinction rate." This is how many species normally shuffle off their mortal coils and end up only a memory in the Burgess Shale. The cause of this extinction? Us.

When I was a kid, the world had Baiji river dolphins, western black rhinoceroses, Pyrenean Ibex, golden toads, and Javan tigers. Finn, who is eight, will grow up in a world in which those species no longer exist.

Since 1950, the climate crises have experienced a boom. We've added 100 parts per million of carbon to the atmosphere—something that hadn't been accomplished in 650,000 years. This melts the ice caps. Sea levels rose about six inches during that past 100 years. The rate of sea levels rising during the past ten years has doubled. The top ten warmest years of the past 135 years occurred during the past twelve years. Things are heating up. Due to the carbon dioxide in the atmosphere produced by the industrial revolution, the earth's oceans are 30 percent more acidic.

These are all statistics that we know—corroborated by dozens of journalistic and scientific sources. Search for "biodiversity threats" and you'll find the *Wall Street Journal*, The International Union for Conservation of Nature, and the Harvard T. H. Chan School of Public Health agreeing that the threat to biodiversity is the major concern in the world, threatening every person on the globe. The sources all agree that rampant development and resource extraction—both of which destroy habitats—are the leading causes of all this environmental chaos.

What is an environmental educator to do?

If your head is spinning because of all the facts, figures, and sheer over-whelmingness of the information above, imagine how an eight-year-old feels confronted with the same data. Not only is it difficult to understand the sheer scale of what we've done to our planet through resource extraction, climate change, pollution, and population growth, but it's also complicated and frus-tratingly hopeless. If an eight-year-old *could* grasp the significance of what we've done to alter our planet in the past fifty years, they'd have the right to shoot spitballs into the face of every adult they see. We deserve it.

In addition, the way in which we approach educating students about the precarious position we've put ourselves in on this planet often depend on the same institutional structures that got us into this mess. Oftentimes, the approaches used to ameliorate the effect development has had is simply dif-ferent kinds of development—large-scale stormwater projects are undertaken to mitigate the effect of runoff from acres of pavement. We build *things* to fix the problems *things* created.

To educate kids about the radical decline of biodiversity, or the importance of sharply reducing the extraction of resources for material development, schools and teachers will need to rethink how education plays a role in shap-ing children's beliefs about their connection to the natural world. Students sitting in bean bag chairs playing "environmental education" games like Clim'way, Recycle City, and Planet Science on an iPad isn't going to cut it.

One of the aims of compulsory, public education has often been stated to be the creation of good citizens. This is something even the shortsighted folks who designed the Common Core apparently agree with, since the only required reading in the Core is the Declaration of Independence. If this is true—that we want our schools to create competent, informed citizens to help steer the ship in the coming generations, then an understanding of the rapid decline of biodiversity and the destruction caused by human development on a global scale should be priority number one. But it isn't happening.

Taking kids outdoors into unstructured environments may help. The way that we interact with the denizens of the woods—the birds, voles, skunks, bugs, and the rest—can determine how well we are able to protect them. Going out, into nature, and making contact with the creatures out there can be a way for us to build rapport with other species, to come to some understand-ing of their lives and wants.

THE WISDOM OF WOODY

Finn and I found the woodpecker in the woods while walking the dog. It was one of the big pileated ones—the size of a crow with a shock of red feathers on its head. It flapped weakly along the ground, the dog sniffing curiously after it while its mate circled through the trees over us, calling out.

I wrapped it in a blanket and brought it home. Once it was covered in darkness of the blanket, it stopped struggling and making sounds. I put it in an emptied out plastic recycling bin and covered the top with the blanket. The bird lay on the bottom, silent. It seemed badly hurt or very sick.

I went inside and called around to find a wildlife rehabilitator and left messages with enough folks that I hoped someone would call back soon. I went out to check on the woodpecker.

I pulled back the blanket from the top of the recycling bin. The bird lay crouched in the corner, defensively, eyes wide open. It looked at me in a way that I had never been looked at before. This was a wild animal, and its gaze was intense. It wasn't the beseeching look of my dog or the aloof, calm look of my cat. It was wild; it asked for no quarter and expected none. Truly, I've never seen anything like it.

There was a raw, primal understanding there, but also this look of realism. It was completely present, and as the bird's eyes stared, unblinking, up at me, I was overcome with the understanding that this was a living creature, full of all the energies that I am. It wanted to live, as all wild things do. It didn't expect any favors from me, and wasn't asking for any. There was no fear—only spring-like tension.

The amount of time we spend in nature extends to how we view ourselves as just one species among many on the planet. Direct, unmediated experience with other animals is vital to developing and understanding of our relationship with the natural world—and our efforts to protect it.

In April 2016, Frans de Waal—a primatologist whose career includes the publication of many vital books about our close evolutionary cousins, monkeys and apes—wrote an essay for the *New York Times* (the essay came out of the studies he presents in a book called *Are We Smart Enough to Know How Smart Animals Are?*) in which he addressed a common bias in the biological sciences: anthropomorphism. De Waal's argument was that the "scientific" approach of scientists to separate animal behavior from human behavior is ill-informed and possibly shortsighted.

He uses the example of tickling a chimpanzee and notes how they respond with laughter and the same giddiness a child would. Normally, scientists wouldn't call the response of the chimp happiness or playfulness; they'd categorize the chimp's laughter as "pant-hoots" as De Waal points out. Anthropomorphism isn't deadly, De Waal asserts, for the simple reason that *we are animals*. Intensely creative, complex, and sophisticated animals, sure, but animals nonetheless.

De Waal invented a new term to categorize the way many scientists try to separate animal behavior from human behavior. *Anthropodenial* is the refusal to accept that humans are on the same continuum of apes and monkeys, mollusks and cuttlefish. We're a species among millions of other species, and when we separate ourselves as distinctly as we do, we run into any number of issues. The fact is that we needed to create some cognitive distance from animals in order to rationalize the way we use them for labor, food, and livelihood. You don't want to eat your cousin and wear their skin as a hat, after all.

The Judeo-Christian tradition addresses this through scriptures that clearly delineate animals from humans. Indigenous peoples who profess a more nuanced view of animals have elaborate—or at least honest—rituals they perform upon killing animals for food or materials. Culturally in the west, we've taken anthropodenial to its extreme, placing animals in an entirely different ideological category than ourselves.

Unfortunately, schools have followed the example of religious instruction and the Judeo-Christian tradition. Our students are way out of touch with the rest of the creatures that share this planet with us.

I was flying on a plane recently and a young kid—maybe nine, ten years old—was playing a video game on an iPad in the row in front of me. It was "Hungry Shark Evolution," a game developed by Future Games of London. It features a shark swimming through levels, munching on fish and collecting "treasure" in the form of shells. The shark develops more and more strength as levels are completed, devouring everything from octopus to scuba divers, each attack accompanied by a little cloud of blood in the water.

There's a whole snarl of interesting ideas here. The gamification of our kids' culture and the slack-jawed screen-time zeitgeist, to name two. But for me watching the kid play the game as his mom scrolled through her iPhone brought up the question of how we're approaching teaching our kids and students about the creatures with whom we're living on this planet.

When I was eighteen I took an Outward Bound trip as a student—an experience I found so transformative it would lead me to work for OB later and sail a wooden boat around the Florida Keys. During the final few days we participated in an open water swim. As I chugged along through the water, I swam directly over a nurse shark. Nurse sharks can grow up to ten feet, but this one was smaller—maybe five, six feet long. I must have startled it with my sluggish and awkward thrashing because it scooted off right underneath me as I swam over it. The water between the mangrove islands we were swimming in was only about eight to ten feet deep. That shark was close.

It scared me. Deeply. I knew, after the shark had shot off, that it was probably harmless—after all, it was trying to escape me and it was clear it just wanted to put space between us, a notion I readily agreed with. But still. A shark. And there I was swimming above it, by myself, the boat a half mile away.

Environmental education needs to align itself not with the current mode of instruction as practiced in the classroom, but with a more radical, direct, unmediated interaction with the outdoor world. The stakes for teaching students the value of biodiversity, the importance of conservation, and the effect of development have never been higher. The clearest route to fostering the kind of deep, nuanced understanding of the natural world is to experience it firsthand.

BECOMING BADGERS

The separation from the natural world most of our indoor schools suffer is debilitating and deadly to our students understanding of other species, and detrimental to their desire to save them. "In our estrangement from nature we have severed our sense of the community of life and lost touch with the experience of other animals," writes Carl Safina in his book on animal cognition and emotion, *Beyond Words*.

It is in these moments that we can engage our students in a direct, nonmediated understanding of the other creatures with whom we share this planet. The consequences of this understanding—or lack thereof—are profound. The future of biodiversity and the other creeping, crawling denizens of our planet depends on teachers fostering a sense of awe and wonder in our students concerning animals in the natural world. Getting them outdoors in the wild can do this. David Neiwert's book, *Of Orcas and Men,* puts it thus:

> Profoundly humbling experiences are good for our souls: those knee-knocking, gut-emptying, jaw-dropping, life-altering moments when you come flat up against the reality that we are each, no matter how big our egos or incomes, insignificant flesh-specks fortunate enough to be alive in this grand universe, those moments such as when we stay up late to see the Milky Way on a summers night in the Rockies, or stand agape at the edge of the grand canyon or an erupting volcano in Hawaii, or watch the birth of our own child. Of all these, there are few as deeply affecting as having an encounter in the wild with one of nature's premier meat-eaters, and of these, none are as profound as having a five-ton killer whale with a towering dorsal fin come looming toward your kayak out of the fog.

There's a rich tradition in Britain of naturalists going to extreme lengths to understand what, exactly, it is like to be an animal. This immersive naturalism is fascinating, and it's surprising how many authors have succumbed to the obsession to figure out a way to clamber into an animal's experience. *The Peregrine* by JA Baker, *Swifts in a Tower* by David Lack—there's a whole slew of British nature writers who try to find their way into the lives of animals. But most recently, Charles Foster's book, *Being a Beast*, has redefined the way we can think about animals—and by animals, I mean ourselves.

Foster's book is tart, laconic, and piercingly funny. The book's structure is straightforward; Foster tries to live the life of a badger, fox, otter, deer, and swift. He digs holes like a badger and eats earthworms, swims naked like an otter, and scavenges the streets of London like an urban red fox. The result is a remarkable work of research, memoir, and adventure, all of which combine to make an interesting philosophical treatise on how we view the other citizens of the world.

Foster writes that most nature writing to this point has been about "striding colonially around, describing what they see from six feet above the ground." In his book, he seeks to reverse that trend and spends a fair amount of text chasing after some wiggly ideas that are difficult to grasp. In particular, Foster is intent on bringing into focus the way our relationships with animals are "intimate," have been, are, and will be. And, how that intimacy filters through much of how we engage with the animal world. Shamans are more apt teachers, one gathers from Foster's book, than environmental educators. Shamans, at least, don't pretend that we aren't in conversation with animals.

These texts can help us pinpoint what, exactly, we are meant to do with outdoor education as it relates to popularized ideas like sustainability, environmental ethics, nature studies, biology, and their ilk. The challenge of the outdoor educator is to get rid of the insulating way that students are ensconced in their worlds through jargon, walls, and institutionally codified presentations of the natural world. What is needed is full immersion—perhaps not actually in a badger hole, as Foster demonstrates, but in such a way as to bring animal's experiences of "selfness" to light. Only in this way can we hope to educate our students and children about the preciousness of life—and the importance of saving it.

It is, at first, a strange idea: a science teacher asking students to crawl through the tall grass, slinking about like a bobcat trying to find nesting birds to eat. The picture gets even odder if we fast-forward the children's age in our imagination. Could we do this with middle schoolers, high school students, college sophomores? This certainly doesn't come from a place of rectitude or shyness. Any teacher worth their salt has leapt about in front of their students, essentially making an ass out of themselves if it serves to bring about understanding. I think the real uncomfortableness of this scenario is our adopting the posture, behavior, and actions of animals. We have so ingrained in our Judeo-Christian culture that animal behaviors are "lower" or more "base" that we've become inured to our estrangement from animals. Animals are—as Foster points out—close relatives, evolutionarily speaking. He writes:

It is a mere 30 million years—the blink of a lightly lidded eye on an earth whose life has been evolving for 3.4 thousand million years—since badgers and I shared a common ancestor. Go back just 40 million years before that, and I share my entire family album not only with badgers but with herring gulls.

All the animals in this book are pretty close family. That's a fact. If it doesn't seem like that, our feelings are biologically illiterate. They need reeducation.

This "reeducation" is what we can do by infusing our lives, our schools, and our teaching with this sort of approach Foster promulgates; deep, meaningful immersion in the natural world for the sake of knowing animals, not in bits of information or as taxonomical categories, but as creatures with wants and needs and lives not terribly unlike our own. It is only once we do this—through embracing a conviction that playing out in the woods like an otter can grace us with a higher level of understanding than any classroom experience ever will—that we will learn to talk to animals again.

And only then can we save them.

Chapter 8

Are You Experienced?

One night on a backpacking trip in the southern Sierra I hung food in a "bear-bag," a pack filled with freeze-dried noodles, granola bars, and other camping victuals, high in a tree from a horizontal branch far from the trunk. It hung suspended above the ground and, hopefully, out of reach of hungry black bears. By the time I finished, it was dark. I headed back to my tent, and only a few minutes had passed when I was startled by a sound from the direction of the bear-bag.

"*Fwooomp!*"

I turned and there, not ten feet away, was a black bear with our food bag in its teeth.

Its eyes reflected yellowish-orange in the beam of my headlamp. The bear whirled, gripping the bag in its teeth, and with incredible speed, galloped off into the darkness. I heard it splash heavily across a stream behind our camp. It was an *experience* I don't think I'll ever forget.

Experiential learning is holistic. It educates the mind and body, but also teaches us interpersonal skills, instructs us in ethics, increases our capacity for grit, and fosters compassion and empathy. Personal development is the unavoidable dividend of experiential education, as is the opportunity for genuine self-reflection. Unlike more narrow ways of learning, outdoor education has both the cultivation of abstract reasoning and the practical application of skills and abilities.

What did I learn in our escapade with the bear? Well, since then, I've learned to be more careful with my food when camping, but the experience fostered understanding that was also more complicated and compelling than that. In reporting my experience to the local rangers afterward, I learned that making food available—even inadvertently—could embolden the bear and make it a problem animal. They may have to remove, or even shoot, such an animal, and now my actions were directly connected to the tangled knot of wildlife management and the difficulties faced in maintaining access for lumbering dolts like me to the outdoors.

Through that experience, I reflected on consequences, on ethics, and had a very real sense of my own mortality. I came to a series of realizations as we tromped our way through the High Sierra over the next few days. I was a visitor in this landscape, just as I would be a visitor in a foreign country. I had to abide by the customs, rules, and culture of the world I was in. I truly learned from the experience, and while the lessons weren't the sort that would fit tidily on a worksheet, they were lasting and transforming.

Experiential learning doesn't have to take such drastic, clear-cut forms, however. Any learning, as long as the learner is engaged and *active participation*, rather than *passively absorbing*, can be considered experiential. Interestingly, it is often the intellectual projects that are the most clearly derived from experience versus pure passive absorption, despite the fact that those projects may appear to be non-experiential. At times, the benefits of allowing students and children to explore their own relationships and themselves outdoors without the interference of adult-centered pedagogy is the most valuable type of learning that can occur.

This is not an endorsement of *Lord of the Flies*–type situations, where teachers hurl kids out into the wilderness to run amok and bash each other over the head with rocks. Nor is it similar to the qualities in programs like girl/boy scouts—organized, institutionalized experiences overtly designed to foster some moral code or directly orchestrated with some character-building goals in mind. Rather, experiential education of this ilk is what happens when we allow schools to develop experiences for students that allow for collaborative, self-initiated experiences for students that allow for their participation in decision making and do so without the usual regulatory influence of four walls and a clock on the wall.

One of the goals of education is to imbue learners with the ability to "know thyself," a concept originally developed by Plato. But what, exactly, does that mean within an educational context? For teachers, it comes down to creating experiences that offer students the chance to navigate understanding on their own terms. It is empowering for children when teachers help them develop the ability to assign meaning to their lives; to define a narrative based not on ticking off boxes or prescribed educational achievement, but one based on the development of self. One of the ways imaginatively projecting themselves into the outdoors helps children learn is that it encourages the creation of a self-mythology that provides agency and empowerment. The skill required to stop and notice things—to be mindful of the present, themselves, and others.

DEVELOPING THE PERSONALITY PORTFOLIO

If you work in education, you know that some of the most generous, kind, insightfully sensitive people hold PhDs, master's degrees, and other symbols of advanced education. Conversely, you probably know some highly educated people that lack the niceties of well-calibrated social skills, and suffer from ignorance, pride, and can be disagreeable. The conclusion we can draw from this is that education does not necessarily make us better people.

Why is that? I mean, shouldn't it? Regardless of discipline, shouldn't most study—from kindergarten through doctorates—confront questions of ethics, empathy, and justice? One would think, and while many do, the fact is that any attempts at molding students into more confident, compassionate, and benevolently gracious humans are at best ancillary to the aims of most educational objectives.

By "better" people what we're talking about is advancing our *personal development*. Personal development is different than physical or intellectual development. In fact, personal development is exactly what it sounds like: the progress of self and identity along a continuum toward a more whole and complete person. One could argue that the more "developed" a person is in this sense, the more capable they are of reflecting on and understanding themselves, the people around them, their communities, and the world in such a way that it gives their actions and beliefs agency toward proactive change for the betterment of the earth and its inhabitants. This is true for the economist, teacher, weather forecaster, barista, athlete, and police officer.

The work of personal development rests in the ability to engage in self-reflection in such a way that a clearer understanding of "self" in relation to "other" becomes clear. For instance, a good self-reflective scenario within this continuum is for a white, straight, middle-class male (ahem, guilty as charged) to reflect on what it might be like to be black, or a woman, or a recent Syrian refugee and also have to look for a job. What must that feel like—what emotions and thoughts would that produce?

An overly simplified example, to be sure. But it's difficult to understand even those closest to us, let alone people who come from vastly diverse backgrounds, but personal development is all about trying to anyway. We ask questions, imagine scenarios. We read, analyze, and think. We identify how we actually might have some stuff in common with the Syrian refugee. We try to bridge gaps through understanding.

It's a tricky business, and personal development usually gets talked about in reference to therapy and counseling, or perhaps with younger students. There seems to be a major drop-off somewhere in adolescence, whereby once we reach adulthood—unless we work in particular educational or social service sectors—*personal development* is no longer a priority and takes a backseat to *professional development*.

There are some teachers within education who do a masterful job of imbuing their lesson plans and practice with a personal development ethos. This isn't some narrow religious definition of morality, however, but rather a tacit understanding of the effect that a teacher's understanding of self in relation to others can have on students—being capable of manifesting a culture in the classroom that fosters a sense of collaboration and community. Being compassionate. To move the needle on fundamental characteristics of students—their generosity, patience, and tolerance—has more to do with *who teachers are*, how they comport themselves in the thousand quotidian moments of their teaching lives, rather than any overarching pedagogical philosophy.

Many teachers, myself included, struggle with the content, wrestle with the strictures of standardized curricula, and essentially just try to keep our heads above water. It can feel like there's very little time for working on personal development when you're trying to teach a room full of hormonally charged little miscreants.

That's where outdoor experiences come into play.

For instance, struggling up a mountain pass and coming face to face with a bear makes you think in particular of your own mortality. You adjust and fine-tune values, reassess your relation to the natural world, and think about your own role in life in a way that can resonate for quite some time. Having these types of experiences, particularly within large chunks of time, allows for students—and let's face it, adults, too—to develop a clearer understanding of ourselves.

In day-to-day interactions, teachers probably don't aid students in personal development all that much. It's not for lack of trying, but the traditional classroom just simply isn't conducive to the kind of experiential problem-based scenarios that call upon teachers to develop a sense of self, others, and community in a proactive way. But outdoor experiences are different. Outdoor experiences are inherently challenging. They push teachers up against very real and concrete personal limitations: physical strength, the ability to work with others, aptitude in getting a fire started, building a tent, cooking food, predicting the weather, and staying warm and dry, just to name some of the most basic requisite skills.

But these outdoor experiences also offer a more internal, abstract personal development; being in these unstructured wilderness environments and pushing their way through landscapes allow teachers and students to tune in to their interior voice. All the nagging concerns, anxieties, and struggles seem to have a way of percolating to the surface during a woodsy trek. Beyond that, teachers and students out and about in the natural world are constantly put in situations that don't just test their mettle and moxie, but their compassion, generosity, and kindness—and they are repeatedly given the chance to better themselves in these instances through thoughtful reflection on the needs of others and even their *own* needs.

The truth is I mess up all the time. Professionally, personally, artistically, physically. They should have my picture under the dictionary definition of "epic fail." Despite my best intentions, I can be selfish, shortsighted, oblivious to the obvious, forgetful, and straight-up ignorant. When I go outdoors it's not as if those unpleasant characteristics go away, but I am provided with infinite opportunities to revise. To inhabit a different skin. To be better than I am.

Typical work and class scenarios we put our students in reward obedience and yes, intelligence, but also competition, selfishness, and ambition. Being with students outdoors offers a multitude of opportunities for them to turn up the dial on the receptivity they have to others' emotions. It gives them the chance to develop traits and behaviors that have positive social results. The same is true for teachers.

BEWARE OF THE SELF

One of the central tenets of personal development, at least from a psychological perspective, is that only by exploring our own psyche can we truly fulfill ourselves and live a life with meaning. This is what the mid-twentieth-century psychologist Abraham Maslow called "self-actualization." Maslow wrote that fully understanding oneself was the apex of personal development. At least, until he debunked his own theory, realizing that if we all just sit around thinking about actualizing ourselves, we're not really thinking about other people—we're being self-absorbed. He extended his theory to the next stage, "self-transcendence," where we move beyond being focused only on ourselves, but begin to take account of the world around us.

This process can be seen directly when teachers take students outside—an experience that provides rich metaphorical ground for just this kind of development. Students who are overly concerned with themselves—solipsistic and self-involved—rarely last long without a healthy (albeit sometimes rude) reminder from the rest of the crew slogging away up the trail that there are other people in the world, thanks very much, who are also tired, sweaty, and uncomfortable. Personal development must come from within, but being outdoors in challenging, rigorous experiences provides groups of students with multiple opportunities to reflect on not just their own lives, but the way they affect those around them.

Personal development of this kind relies on self-awareness. While "self-awareness" is a term that gets bandied about a fair bit, dialing in on what, exactly, it means and how it relates to personal development will make it clear that outdoor trips such as long overnight treks in the mountains are excellent at fostering just this kind of thinking.

Narrative identity is a term that has been coined to define this type of under-standing, and it relates both to personal development and plays a central role in self-awareness. Dan McAdams, a professor at Northwestern, describes nar-rative identity as "a person's internalized and evolving life story, integrating the reconstructed past and imagined future to provide life with some degree of unity and purpose." McAdams and other researchers' work on narrative iden-tity is helpful in disseminating the effect the outdoors has on the whole student as opposed to more traditionally narrow terms of development, and helpful in looking at the importance of experience in relation to self-awareness.

The concepts behind narrative identity theory are that stories that we tell others about our own lives help to define both who we are, and also give meaning to events that may seem meaningless without the helpful context of a narrative. McAdams calls this "integration," the way we organize thoughts, events, and people in the stories we tell ourselves and other people that help define us. In addition, there have been strong correlations between the abil-ity to tell a good life story about oneself and psychological health; it would appear that individuals who are able to provide a convincing narrative about their own life story have healthy egos and a higher level of self-awareness than those who can't.

Most people love a good story. Some of my own favorite stories involve the outdoors. This is hardly surprising. I like hiking, camping, and canoeing, so clearly I'd enjoy stories about those activities more than, say, someone recounting their heroism in making piles of money in the junk bond mar-ket. Booooring. But beyond that, the outdoors provides such rich materials for these stories. Usually intense or funny, sometimes with a metaphysical, semi-spiritual take on self-awareness, stories of the wilderness abound with *meaning*.

Stories of the outdoors are inclusive. Everyone has some experience, no matter how limited, with the themes of outdoor stories such as being lost, hungry, in the dark, or confronting physical challenges. One of my favorite stories I tell concerning the outdoors is about the time I fell into a latrine in the Colorado Rockies, and every time I tell it I'm reminded that it's not just a funny story, it's relatable. It's real. (It's also really, really gross.)

If a healthy self-awareness can benefit from developing this narrative iden-tity, it follows that providing children with the sorts of experiences that make for good stories is essential. A story about the time they filled out a math worksheet seems a bit dull, really. How can a kid tell that story and make themselves the hero, build empathy, and present a version of themselves that's maybe a bit stronger, or braver, or kinder, than they really are? This isn't just fudging the truth, but an essential part of why narrative identity is so important.

When people offer up versions of themselves as strong (what the researchers call "John Wayne") or kind and caring ("Florence Nightingale"), they provide themselves with a template with which they can make positive transformations in their lives. Taking children outside, into the experientially based world of nature, provides them with the ingredients for great stories. As they tell these stories, again and again, they refine their understanding of self.

McAdams notes that these "redemptive narratives" of overcoming suffering and obstacles are key to developing a positive sense of self. If the job of teachers and parents is to help children develop into competent, kind, and self-aware creatures, taking them outdoors for long periods of time is an essential component.

You should know that I tell that story of the bear all the time. It has become a part of my narrative identity—a chance to relate to people through a time when I was scared, foolish, bumbling. It was a time when I was interacting in the world in a real way. That moment has become interlaced with my understanding of myself.

The outdoors, in addition to providing this rich soil for students to sow their own life stories, also provides teachers with a ton of "teachable moments." In educational circles this is sometimes referred to as *incidental teaching*. Essentially, it's stopping during an experience and using it to provide insight into some broader concept.

As a pedagogical approach, it's most helpful in trying to get students to understand abstract concepts like compassion and empathy. How are teachers to teach students to value and protect the experiences of others? To ensure that they care for those around them who are suffering? Educators can't just *make* students care—they have to model it. Teachers must provide them with moments where they can enact their own version of empathy and receive the rewards: gratitude, social standing, and praise. Being in the outdoors in unstructured environments provides so many of these moments. "Jimmy, how do you think Darla felt when you smacked her in the head with that branch?" That sort of thing.

Compassion and empathy cannot be taught as abstract concepts—they must be lived. Incidental teaching moments are valuable in allowing students to gain an understanding of the order of events, their import, and meaning. In addition, being outdoors for extended periods of time gives teachers the chance to explore the development of self with their students during moments of awe, collaboration, frustration, suffering, and joy. Experience in nature gives us these moments.

ON LEARNING AND FRIENDSHIP

There are many ingredients that go into successful teaching that produce rewarding and fulfilling learning experiences. In fact, learning is so highly integrated into our lives that many of the most important factors that lead to knowledge acquisition, personal development, skill building, and academic ability lay outside the boundaries of traditional schooling. The sort of nurturing and support received as infants and young children; families' socioeconomic standing; health, community, and culture all play a role in how individuals end up approaching education as learners. But teachers arguably play one of the largest roles, and there are countless inspiring stories of teachers who've helped students succeed despite struggles outside the classroom. With 180 days of school per year on average, and anywhere from six to eight hours spent in the classroom or engaged in education per day, the people standing in front of the room *matter*.

And it's not just their training and experience that matters, either. The relationship between a student and teacher is essential to fostering learning, and that relationship pays dividends if it's based on trust.

One of the challenges that face positive student–teacher relationships is inequity. Teachers occupy a position of such arbitrary authority that the very nature of positive relationships—a give-and-take flexibility that allows for change and equal engagement between two independent but mutually supportive people—is difficult to achieve. In fact, the very openness and vulnerability that enables intimate and close relationships could be misconstrued as rather, umm, *icky* in an educational setting. No one wants their kid's kindergarten teacher pouring their heart out to a confused child about their disastrous divorce.

Positive relationships between mutually supportive people become even more difficult when one considers how schools function competitively rather than collaboratively, and through hierarchical authority based on rank, power, and age rather than on consensus built through equal participation and communal decision making. There are courageous examples of these more radical models out there, such as the Philly Free School, where students are as much a part of the decision-making process as the adults. But for tens of millions of kids in public schools, their daily context doesn't necessarily provide the best environment for developing meaningful relationships with their teachers. The fact that they do, and often, is a testament to the power of human relationships and a triumph of teachers everywhere.

It may be helpful here to state the argument plainly: the relationship between a student and teacher is the most crucial factor in developing motivated, explorative, confident, curious learners. The equation is, perhaps, a bit lopsided: students who lack positive relationships with their teachers *may* learn; those with those types of relationships *will* learn.

The literature about the importance of teaching in this relationship-based way (as opposed to teaching in a resolutely authoritarian or results-oriented manner, for example) is persuasive in that it offers key insights into just how vital it is to think about forming positive relationships with students.

Studies have shown repeatedly that students who have positive relationships with their teachers perform better academically. This seems like a bit of rather intuitive common sense to most of us; of course they learn better surrounded by caring people. Duh. But the research brings some interesting points to bear on the how and why of it.

Christopher Murray, chair of the Special Education and Clinical Sciences department at the University of Oregon, noted in a 2005 report that "closeness-trust with teachers made particularly strong contributions to school adjustment." The report also notes that student engagement was significantly affected by the relationships teachers had with their students. This is key: the closeness felt inspires motivation, and a lack of openness inhibits learning.

And yet in the contemporary standards-driven climate, how much attention is paid to training teachers to develop these relationships, to foster a culture of inclusiveness and trust, both in regard to classroom dynamics, but perhaps more importantly in their one-on-one relationships with students? The answer, unfortunately, is not much. Research from the *Journal of Educational Psychology* noted that "teachers receive very little or no preparation in building successful alliances with parents or supportive and warm relationships with students."

Academic success doesn't exist in a vacuum; positive social conditions play a significant role in predicting student outcomes as well. Researchers from Virginia Tech applied social capital theory to the classroom and found some intriguing results. Students and teachers build social capital by caring for one another and having positive interactions and expectations—being caring for a student and encouraging and expecting them to do well build social capital, as do demonstrating acceptance and creating empathetic relationships with individual students.

Students who are accepted and cared for by teachers are more likely to be accepted and cared for by their peers. This seems like a no-brainer, yet in looking at the interactions of the classroom how often are teachers predisposed to think negatively of a student, or substitute some hackneyed version of "tough love" rather than genuine caring? Admittedly, sometimes it's tough. That whining, needy student who won't let you be, or the aloof, jaded guy in the back row who tries to wear sunglasses the first day—those sorts can be an annoying handful and test our patience. The evidence seems to strongly suggest that fostering open, trusting caring relationships with students motivates them and improves academic performance and social conditions in the classroom.

But how do we achieve this in daily practice? Are we supposed to be just "nice" to our students, and then *WHAM* they're doubling majoring in political science and biochemistry at Harvard?

The problem in my limited experience is that just being the nice, cool guy who's friendly to everyone lowers the bar. Deliberately building positive relationships isn't the same as just kicking back and handing out skittles. I wish it were that easy. Do that, and you're as likely to be mowed down as a softie as have positive results.

In order to create these relationships—build trust, break down walls, and be open with students—teachers have to be intentional about their interactions and create experiences wherein that trust and openness can be nurtured. The classroom presents teachers with circumstances that seem abstract and arbitrary. A teacher places a student up in the front of the room to help them pay better attention and the student perceives the effort as punishment. Only by initiating relationships outdoors in unstructured environments can education offer students and teachers straightforward, practical, tangible models for building exactly the type of positive relationships that are such good predictors of student success.

Once outdoors, teachers are given so many chances for a thousand small gestures of kindness. Often, on longer trips in the backcountry or while rock climbing, for instance, the trust built between students and teachers isn't some abstract, conceptual thing. Teachers, for instance, could have students on belay, anchoring them, keeping them aloft. For those of us who have participated in these outdoor activities, it isn't unusual that we directly entrust one another with our lives.

Daniel Deronda, Eliot's fictional hero, seeks to impart meaning in his life. He does so through relationships, first with Mirah Lapidoth and then with Mordecai. In both cases there are a series of experiences that guide those relationships toward mutual trust, friendship, learning, a sense of shared purpose—even love. So too do teachers seek some meaning in what they do, some reckoning by which they navigate days filled with administrative demands, grumbling parents, asinine standards, and compulsive institutional expectations. That meaning is derived from the bond they have with students—the joyful, electric give-and-take that occurs while teaching and learning. And outdoors, as teachers and students help each other over storm-downed trees; lose the trail only to find it again; share a granola bar, and pass the sunscreen around the groundwork is laid for trust. The rapport necessary for authentic learning is best built under the pines out in the open air.

When all's said and done, learning can be boiled down to the dance two people engage in when one leads and one follows. But as any dancer will tell you, the trust implicit in pulling off a successful waltz is so central to the experience of dancing that without it the dance is doomed. And though we use words like "respect" and "relationship" and all kinds of language to distance ourselves from the matter at hand, what we're talking about when we talk about learning is friendship.

Within the circle of this friendship we find the roots of learning. And this learning is sometimes born of a hand offering to help you up a steep grade, a swallow of water to soothe a parched throat. The act of learning and teaching is two souls in a darkened forest, sharing one headlamp that bounces a giddy path through the night to find a tent, and, finally, at the end of a long, sweaty, challenging day, they gratefully crawl into sleeping bags, zipping out the darkness, secure in the knowledge of trust and shared experience, to fall asleep and wake up the next day to become who they were meant to be.

Chapter 9

The Right to Outdoor Play

When I was twenty-five years old, I helped start and run a small, independent elementary and middle school in Los Angeles. My young age, in addition to a pretty immature sensibility combined with a rather puerile sense of humor, meant that there was a lot of roughhousing. The boys and I would—quite literally—spend entire afternoons horsing around. Bruises bloomed (mostly on me). If you've ever been ganged up on by a pack of fourteen-year-olds, you know what I'm talking about. Bodies banged and fell and flew about, and hilarity and good times ensued. It was the sort of play that would send a bureaucratic "risk assessor" into hyperventilation. To us it was just fun.

Our rough play was, in part, a way to use physical touch to process trust and develop a sense of one another. To be close to each other without having to necessarily be emotionally vulnerable, which can be hard for boys that age, was something that helped us ground ourselves. Headlocks and noogies and sucker punches were the way we showed love.

Americans are—in comparison with other cultures—touch-averse. Those who study proxemics, which is the physical distance between bodies in a given environment, have found that Americans are rather stuffy about touch. We're a bit uptight compared to Europeans or Asians. One period when this is *not* true is childhood, during which children are constantly touching, grabbing, tussling, and reaffirming trust through gentle grooming, simple proximity, or horseplay.

One game we played at the little school I worked at was called "Hong Kong Basketball," an homage to the Kung Fu movies of Jackie Chan that we loved. It was basketball—sort of—combined with an MMA cage match. You'd try to get the ball in the hoop, but other players would be punching, grabbing, and body checking you. After a while, the game devolved into a hilariously fun and rough free-for-all, ball forgotten.

At first, the female students didn't play. One day Megan, a thirteen-year-old girl, jumped into the fray. I did treat her differently. The boys I'd fling about, but I wouldn't do that with Megan. She *wanted* to play, though. She wanted the very real physical release that comes from rough and tumble fun, but I wasn't comfortable engaging with her in that way.

Unconsciously, I promoted the age-old stereotype that girls are more fragile than boys, that they don't find fun (and prosocial, as well as personal developmental dividends) in rough play. Oddly, I thought that by not letting her play—by treating her by some different set of rules based on her gender—I was establishing trust between us. In fact, rough play is *the* way to establish rapport and trust among most social species. Instead of a gesture of respect or thoughtfulness, my unwillingness to engage Megan physically was reinforcing all the negative stereotypes that have been passed down for far too long: girls are weaker, girls are fragile. Girls should be treated differently.

Megan was having none of my bullshit.

"It's not fair!" she said. There was an edge to her voice, a barely suppressed rage that hid beneath the more common adolescent indignation. "What?" I asked, as the knot of punching, kicking boys untangled themselves and flopped about, smiling and catching their breath. "You treat me differently because I'm a girl." There it was. The moment sticks out in my memory in hyper-definition, like an airbrushed tiger on a carnival T-shirt. She was right.

Part of my hesitation sprung from quasi-conservative social values I'd absorbed. I was a twenty-five-year-old man. She was a thirteen-year-old girl. We all know the stories and how the power dynamic of an older male and a young girl has played out in certain situations in the past. But we've also been educated to believe that rough and tumble play between people separated by age and gender in any arrangement is verboten. And it's understandable. I'm sure I'd have had a few questions if my daughter came home describing how she'd had so much fun wrestling with her older male teacher on the floor during lunch. But it's exactly this fear that deprives girls of what they need.

It further perpetuates the misogynist myth that female bodies are weak; that girls and women's bodies are meant to be looked at and venerated as abstract ideas rather than used as powerful tools for work and play. In fact, girls have a *right* to play—female's right to play rough is aligned with all the work done by women's movements for the past century. It is one of the most deeply entrenched social discriminations—the treatment of women and girls as physically less than men. We all know the stories and statistics. Around Megan's age, girls begin to have any number of deep concerns about their bodies and looks thanks in part to our completely warped culture of celebrated celluloid anorexia and unattainable digitally altered beauty. Author Gerard Jones writes:

> When girls don't feel free to play at open aggression, their desire to play with power and conflict don't go away but take other forms. Lenore Terr noted "After they've abandoned rough-and-tumble play, girl's social play can become extremely aggressive. Games about inclusion and exclusion, social competition and defeat, express a great deal of aggression."

I wasn't helping Megan face the challenges of adolescence as a girl. The best thing I could've done was let her put me in a headlock or gut-punch me.

WRESTLING WITH THE OUTDOORS

The artificial divide that exists between the genders in the indoor, socially constructed, institutionally regulated, and pop-culturally informed classroom is bolstered due to the very way classrooms operate on traditionally patriarchal, or at the very least hierarchical, grounds. The outdoors—especially the outdoors as an unstructured, collaboration-inducing, flexible group experience—does a good job at eroding the harmful distinctions kids (and teachers) draw between the genders.

Note that I use the term "gender" here purposefully instead of "sex." Biological differences aside, the issue of how we treat traditionally construed genders lies in cultural attitudes, not because of their biology, so when we speak of "girls" and "boys," we mean individuals possess and exhibit behaviors that would fall within those traditionally (though incomplete) cultural descriptions.

Unstructured, outdoor, experiential learning provides an excellent forum to challenge these notions of gender divides that plague schools. Because success in the outdoors requires such a great number of various skills—including teamwork, strength, agility, intelligence, empathy, planning, foresight—the individuals who do well often surprise even those of us who've spent a considerable amount of time outdoors. The supersmart classroom geek may wither under the challenges of the woods; the classically cocksure bully may be afraid of the dark (they almost always are); the quiet wallflower turns out to have a knack for endurance and woodcraft beyond imagining, and the superdistracted class clown is able to flit about, helping carry a pack here, set up a shelter there, and find harmony with the endless space and exploration offered by the wilderness.

One of the problems is that the issue of play is often demoted to a lessor position compared to learning. And the *right* to play outdoors, though widely recognized as a part of childhood, is rarely given the same weight as other concerns. Megan's need for physical play, and her desire to be treated equally, might be tossed aside as minor concerns in the face of other more seemingly important educational challenges.

#FIRSTWORLDPROBLEMS

Over the past few years, social media have abounded with comments, posts, and critiques using the hashtag #firstworldproblems. The idea behind this internet trend is that concerns, complaints, and whining done by privileged groups—that is, western, affluent, usually white people—existed in a subcategory. Real suffering, or problems, exist only within individuals from other parts of the world that, according to the ideology behind the hashtag, had a more legitimate claim on pain than those in the developed world.

Articulating the conceptual nuances of this idea requires some untangling. It isn't the hashtag itself that is troubling. How privileged western people (like myself) frame their experiences against a global backdrop of "have and have-nots," while an interesting sociopolitical and philosophical problem suggesting an oddly passive aggressive, shame-based agenda is not the primary sticking point from an educational philosophy point of view. It is an issue that can misdirect the conversation around taking kids of all sorts up into the mountains in a way that could prove to be detrimental.

Hackneyed social media phrases like #firstworldproblems can undermine the importance of outdoor experiences for educational and personal development. They can be made to seem unimportant and light-weight. In short: isn't arguing for more time outdoors for kids in the United States at a time when millions of Syrian refugees crowd the borders of Europe; widespread corruption undermines democracies in Haiti and elsewhere; and 2.8 billion people worldwide live on less than two dollars a day according to the UN a kind of elitist, first world problem? Why argue for more time to play outdoors when starvation, war, and human trafficking are extant the world over? The line of reasoning could be articulated thus: who cares about "less screen, more green" in times like these?

The Universal Declaration of Human Rights (UDHR) is the formational document through which much of the work being done around the world by governments, NGOs, and individuals in development is based. Drafted by members of the UN General Assembly in 1948, among other things it includes rights to privacy, property, and legal protection, as well as prohibiting slavery and torture. The document acts as a blueprint of sorts, laying out the foundation for a democratic, safe, progressive society.

One of the observations made about the UDHR is that it represents a picture of life that is particularly western, industrialized, privatized, and capitalistic—thereby negating other means of governance, cultures, and technologies (or lack thereof) that may exist outside of the boundaries the authors of the document prescribe. Nonetheless, it is an essential document that acts as a baseline for the international community to use to do the vital work of fighting for human rights. Here are the rights, the UDHR claims, which we need to have just, stable societies.

It's hard to contest the rights listed. Rights to education, social security, and health care in case of illness, and peaceful assembly are pretty good ideas—essential attributes to any society that hopes to have some degree of safety and freedom for its citizens. But nowhere in the UDHR does it state that children have the right to play outside. Taken as a whole, the absence of access to nature as a means of education and leisure (leisure is listed as a right but one that is uncontextualized) suggests that, as far as human rights go, there is a hierarchy. Ensuring that children have access to food, shelter, education, and health care seems to be more important than them climbing trees or catching frogs.

"What looks like a hierarchy is actually a web," Adam said. We were hiking through Dogtown, a poison ivy–infested tract of wooded land smack-dab in the middle of Cape Ann in Northern Massachusetts. In the nineteenth century, Dogtown was populated by riffraff and cast-offs, and earned its name due to the packs of feral dogs that populated the scrubby, wrinkled landscape.

Legends and stories abound about Dogtown, everything from witches to hauntings, and today it's a preserved park with a latticed network of trails crisscrossing the heavily wooded hills and valleys. We were there to celebrate Adam's wife's birthday, and as usual our celebration weekend included an excursion into the woods. As Adam and I lagged behind the group, he explained to me that while we see some human rights—education, legal protection—as more important than others, the fact is that human rights are very much interdependent on each other—more like an ecosystem than a hierarchy.

As a human rights scholar and author, Adam had a fascinating take on the relationship access to unstructured time outdoors had to the UDHR. The UDHR, Adam told me, was essentially a list of *rights to the indoors*. It was a document that was designed—after the atrocities of World War II and the Holocaust—to create an even playing field globally, but that playing field rested on assumptions, including the assumed benefits of a westernized, industrialized, and hierarchical society. The right to leisure had more to do with the safety and comfort of the home—the right to leisure is article 24 within the UDHR, the right to "housing" is found within article 25—than getting out for a hike.

As we succeeded in getting thoroughly lost on the spooky, winding trails of Dogtown, Adam asked me to imagine the negation of the rights listed in the UDHR taken to their ultimate conclusion. If, for example, there *was* an article in the UDHR guaranteeing kids the right to access playtime outdoors, the absolute absence of such a right would mean they were locked indoors, all the time. They'd be perpetually imprisoned.

It follows that the right to play outside isn't separate from the right to safety or leisure or education. It is an integral part of all those, an interconnected fiber without which other human rights lack meaning.

I said, "Providing kids with time outdoors—unstructured access to natural environments to play and be imaginative—should be a right for all children."

"That would be the worst thing to happen to the outdoors," Adam said.

Surprised, I asked why.

Adam explained that if *only* kids had the right to the outdoors, and we left adults out of the equation, it would be a flawed right. Because children are, for better or for worse, under the authority and influence of adults, the way we prescribe rights for all people regardless of age matters very much. Human rights need to be comprehensive—not just favor particular groups. I thought about the way outdoor time was negated on a daily basis in the professional world: endless departmental meetings, webinars, focus groups, and conference calls make it difficult for many individuals to benefit from time spent outdoors.

In order to guarantee that all kids get time outside—to grow, to play, to develop empathy, and to use their imagination—we have to ensure that *all* people have a right to the outdoors. The valuing of outdoor experiences for children can't just be an issue for outdoor educators. Parents, governments, and society as a whole need to value outdoor access for everyone.

During the Great Depression, millionaire philanthropist Roger W. Babson hired stonecutters to inscribe inspirational words and phrases on some of the huge, gray, elephantine boulders scattered around the woods of Dogtown. "Help Mother," "Kindness," "Spiritual Power," and "Get a Job" are just a few of the carvings in the massive rocks. As we wended our way out of Dogtown, we passed a smaller rock, on which was carved a single word: "Ideas." I believe one of the ideas we need to visit more often—and with more attention—is the idea of *play*.

PLAY LIKE YOUR LIFE DEPENDS ON IT (BECAUSE IT DOES)

When we think of kids outdoors we usually think of them playing. Chasing one another, building forts, climbing trees, sword fighting with sticks, making mud pies, arguing about the complicated rules of some pretend game.

Understanding the relationship between the outdoors and unstructured play is vital to understanding just why getting children outside into natural environments is so essential for their well-being, their health, and their intellectual, social, and emotional development. But even beyond those crucial factors, understanding outdoor play is necessary in order to delve into the murky waters of self-actualization and the way children begin to develop a sense of individual and social identity.

Play is, perhaps not surprisingly, a behavior that humans share with many other species. Many animals, particularly young mammals, exhibit behavior that is clearly playful. Young bear cubs tumbling and play-fighting, frisky colts kicking up their heels—these acts are part of the same set of traits and behaviors that define human play, particularly human play in young children. But what, exactly, is play?

The field of play research—generally inhabited by psychologists but with a few anthropologists, neuroscientists, and other disciplines thrown in for seasoning—is broad, deep, and endlessly fascinating. And in fact, this very question, "what is play?" has occupied more than a few of these researchers for the past couple of decades.

Drawing distinctions between play-fighting and real fighting, for instance, can be a bit more difficult than one might think at first glance. While by no means the single or most widely accepted definition of play, for the sake of brevity and cohesion it is easiest to go with a definition penned by Scott Eberle, vice president for play studies at The Strong Museum of Play, and author and editor of the *American Journal of Play*. Eberle states that play is "an ancient, voluntary 'emergent' process driven by pleasure that yet strengthens our muscles, instructs our social skills, tempers and deepens our positive emotions, and enables a state of balance that leaves us poised to play some more."

Play is synonymous with the outdoors. The lack of hierarchical structure, the manner in which young children engage with one another and the environment, and the availability of landscapes conducive to pretend or seeking games lend themselves to play. In the outdoors, especially in natural, unstructured environments, play is well-nigh irresistible. In fact, children are so prone to play outdoors that—inclement weather not withstanding—one could argue that the entire purpose of school buildings is to separate kids from the never-ending and satisfyingly distracting opportunities for play that exist outdoors.

The benefits of play go beyond the "strengthening of muscles" and the development of positive emotions. But first, it's important to ask where play comes from. Is it genetic, inherited evolutionarily? Learned? When humans play, we are engaging in one of the oldest (evolutionarily speaking) expressions of emotions—and also developing the highest order of executive functions intellectually. Just how this is possible requires a step back to examine the roots of play, which have much to do with how our species is hardwired, neurologically.

Where play exists neurologically, and how play expresses itself behaviorally in an evolutionary sense are key parts of the puzzle of how play is related to learning. Do brains have different sections, or parts, for cognitive tasks like calculating compound interest and answering questions on a job interview than for engaging in playful activities like perfecting the perfect armpit fart noise and performing a spot-on Sponge Bob impersonation?

As renowned psychologist Jaak Panksepp—a Distinguished Research Professor Emeritus at Bowling Green State University—points out, humans are arguably the most cognitively and behaviorally complex species on the planet. The reasons for this are many: our clever hands with opposable thumbs, our ability to make a wide variety of sounds for communication, our upright stance, and our social communication to name a few. Most of our abilities are that we often think are particularly amazing come from the neocortex, the most recently evolved part of our brain that grows like gangbusters from birth onward in normal development, and gives rise to reading, writing, math, and storytelling—all the stuff of culture.

Surprisingly, play is not associated with all the fancier attributes of the neocortex. It's an older drive, evolutionarily speaking, and thus resides in the organization and interplay of subneocortical brain circuits.

In a paper that addressed the psychobiology of play, Panksepp lays it out for us thus:

> A diversity of ancient genetically coded affective-emotional survival systems emerged progressively in brain evolution: SEEKING, FEAR, RAGE, LUST, CARE, PANIC, or separation distress, and most important for this discussion, social PLAY. Here I capitalize PLAY and other words among these protective and life-supporting "primary-processes" emotional-affective survival networks of the brain-mind to highlight key terminological issues and give this intrinsic mammalian brain process the attention it deserves.

The take-home message is clear: in terms of evolution, *play was necessary for survival*. This is no small point. If play is such an inherent drive—such a fundamental building block of both our behavioral and neurological makeup—then the denial of such a drive could ostensibly lead to drastic results.

When species are denied access to behaviors, environments, and activities that are essential to their functioning, there can be negative consequences. Parrots denied social interaction will pluck out their own feathers because social interaction and the benefits derived from it are central to their evolutionary design. Thus play is with children. But often, the play of children can be viewed as overwhelmingly negative—especially play that has violent themes of guns, death, and warfare.

Not only is play viewed as a "waste" of time (a very old idea that has as much to do with religious restrictions based on biblical notions of "idleness" as a culture of industry and pragmatic activity that is deep in the American tissue), but in contemporary culture it is often viewed inaccurately as a harbinger of behaviors to come. Violently themed play among children is considered to be a harbinger of violent behavior later in life.

KILLING ORCS

I worry—to an annoying degree of anxiety—that I expose Finn to too much violence. As a lifelong fan of Marvel's X Men, Star Wars, and all things Tolkien, our dad–son play is filled with clashing broadswords, the hammered skulls of orcs, sizzling lightsaber strikes, and general bloody melee. Pretend melee, but melee nonetheless.

In fact, it's the sort of play Finn would get admonished for in school. As a family we've reenacted what Finn refers to as the "generator room battle" from Star Wars: Episode I about a million times. In it, a young Obi Wan Kenobi and his master Qui Gon Jinn battle the Sith apprentice Darth Maul. Jinn gets stabbed through the chest, and Kenobi exacts his revenge on the red and black tattooed and horned Maul by cutting the Sith fighter in half and hurling his parts down a huge shaft. Finn, his mother, and I have replayed this drama again and again, taking turns as characters and stabbing and cutting our way through the action. It's wicked violent and crazy fun.

But I wonder, what lessons am I teaching Finn by opening the floodgates to this kind of imaginary play? Am I filling his head with dark images and ideas that will spawn outward, expressing themselves in some horrible way in Finn's adolescence or adulthood?

In his fascinating and compulsively readable book, *Killing Monsters*, author Gerard Jones (mentioned earlier) discusses exactly these issues. As a writer (and father) who has worked in comics and animation, Jones has a unique perspective on why kids actually *need* this kind of violent, rough, and tumble imaginative play. He notes that after the shootings in Columbine, children at the schools he visited to facilitate comics workshops were upset and unsettled. "Kids were jittery that spring," he writes. He goes on to relate that when children immerse themselves in fantasy violence like Pokémon, Dragon Ball Z, or even Star Wars, it provides a much-needed release. "I believe those safe, endlessly repeated trips into fantasy violence played a role in helping a nation of anxious children work through their fears."

On one level, it is clear that play is what teaches young children social rules. Who plays with whom, how rough, and when are the primary building blocks for developing a sense of acceptable social behavior. The benefits of long stretches of outdoor time are inestimable: when children are given the opportunity to engage in free-form play, often roughhousing, they are able to develop the very tools needed later on in life.

Moreover, to deny that children have dark thoughts and the need to work through them places them at great risk. Particularly now, with the prevalence of screens and constant media, children are exposed to visions of violence and complicated ideas of warfare and fear on a daily basis. Rough, outdoor play—for both boys *and* girls—not only allows them the chance to bodily process these realities, but also stabilizes their emotions and allows them to develop self-confidence and an awareness of their own limitations and, perhaps more importantly, the limitations of others.

Rough, outdoor play is more than just a way to pass the time; it is an inviolable right of children around the world.

Chapter 10

Enkidu's Lament

Once students enter middle and high school, outdoor experiences in unstructured natural environments are almost nonexistent, save for a few schools with experiential education programs. Most outdoor time is relegated to athletic fields, which follows many of the same institutional constraints as the school day: gender segregation, age segregation, competition, and socioeconomic favoritism. Even outdoor time in elementary school is often scripted, controlled, and brief.

Part of the issue may be that kids rambling around outside may just look like they're goofing off, but underneath that is a more substantial bias that rests on some pretty deeply ingrained assumptions about "outdoor experiences." In critically examining the basis by which educational systems identify activities that are seen as more positive than others, it seems possible that outdoor play—in the context of contemporary American educational philosophy—is seen as more "primitive" a learning style. This is due to the hierarchy created by western civilization that values indoor, civilized environments that—perhaps inadvertently—reinforce dominant paradigms like racism, sexism, patriarchy, and classism.

Why does education equate outdoor experiences as more primitive and less valuable? This is an age-old prejudice based on a sense of violently guarded superiority on behalf of landowners, as well as a philosophy embraced by colonial powers exploiting less technologically developed regions during the age of exploration. It's worth repeating here: our current system of education is based on the historical models that precede it; those models incorporate structures from colonialism, religious teaching, industrialism, and imperialism. Those with material wealth had to create a system whereby those who owned the land (or actively lived on it, hunting or foraging) were seen as inferior so that there could be a philosophical, religious, or moral ramification for taking the land away, pillaging resources, and subjugating people.

This age-old dualism still exists today. The outdoors is "dirty" and for "play,"' and the indoors somehow more "clean," more refined. This has been true for several hundred years of western history, despite the fact that until recently the indoors were incredibly dirty, at least in terms of breeding epidemics like cholera and other communicable diseases. However, it has been the case for a long time that those who live outside and close to the land are seen as less-civilized, more animal like, and thus in need of education or taming.

Early on, in the very first cities, a mark of superiority had to be bestowed on the indoor dwelling folks, a good example being the dichotomy between Gilgamesh and Enkidu. The ancient Sumerian myth *Gilgamesh*, which dates from around roughly 1200 BCE, is perhaps the earliest story in which a civilized character, Gilgamesh, has to subdue and clean up his wild counterpart, Enkidu. The story of Enkidu and Gilgamesh is an excellent metaphor for how the west has approached ideas surrounding the outdoors—an approach that has been infused in contemporary education, unwittingly or not.

Enkidu begins the story as a hairy half-savage man beast, described in one version of the ancient poem as "rough bodied" with "long hair." Ostensibly Enkidu was created by gods in response to the king's subjects—they prayed to curb the tyrannical habits of Gilgamesh by creating Enkidu to defeat him and teach him some humility, but it's Enkidu who gets subdued. Before his "taming" by Gilgamesh, Enkidu is described thus:

> This Enkidu was innocent of mankind.
> He knew not the cultivated land.
> Enkidu was in the hills with the gazelles -
> They jostled each other
> With all the herds
> He too loved the water-hole.

Gilgamesh's victory in taming Enkidu and bringing him under the civilizing influence is western literature's first example of the triumph of urbanity, the superiority of agriculture and pastoral pursuits, versus more direct, unfettered contact with nature. Within the confines of the story it's seen as a good thing that Enkidu is brought under the tutelage of Gilgamesh to be made into a respectable citizen. But as one of the oldest known stories—one that dates from the creation of the very first city states—this story sets the stage for many of the western world's most central motifs concerning nature versus civilization, including most of the tales in western religion. Beyond that, the very seed of the way in which those who live closely to nature are discriminated against is seen in arguably one of the first stories widely circulated in western culture.

This dynamic of subduing outdoor dwelling races or characters through superior technology, learning, or even ideology can be seen in the biblical story of Adam and Eve—another ancient text that has had an even more pervasive effect in shaping educational institutions. Written over a span of time that overlaps the writing of Gilgamesh, the way the Bible addresses nature—especially in the story of Adam and Eve—has become a central motif in the Judeo-Christian-based allegorical stories that underpin much of western culture.

So important is the story of Adam and Eve, and their expulsion from the Garden of Eden, that it's a shared story of Christians, Muslims, and Jews. Both Jesus of Nazareth and Mohammad can trace their ancestry back to Adam. What happened in the Garden of Eden is a vital story for understanding the most basic and common elements of the shared perspective of the Abrahamic religions, and also the way much of religion—and by extension education—grapples with the idea of nature and human beings' relationship with it.

BIBLICAL HIPPIES

Adam and Eve were created by God to enjoy the Garden of Eden. They cavorted about, naked, eating fruits from the trees and resembling happy hippies on a commune. But, there was a snake in the grass: Satan. Both the Old Testament and the Koran agree on the way Satan figures into the story—a fallen angel, a djinn, basically a creature of supernatural force who has somehow gained the will to go against God.

Adam's responsibilities are clearly delineated by God, as stated in the King James Version of the Bible;

> And the LORD God took the man, and put him into the Garden of
> Eden to dress it and to keep it.
> And the LORD God commanded the man, saying, Of every tree of
> the garden thou mayest freely eat:
> But of the tree of the knowledge of good and evil, thou shalt not eat
> of it: for in the day that thou eatest thereof thou shalt surely die.

Later, God will make Adam a woman from his rib—Eve—and the two will wander naked and blissful through the garden together, snacking on fruits and vegetables and eating what sounds like a very fibrous diet. But Satan—disguised, not very cleverly, as a snake—tempts Eve to eat the forbidden fruit. She does, and suddenly, she and Adam realize their basic sin: nakedness.

> And the eyes of them both were opened, and they knew that they were naked;
> and they sewed fig leaves together, and made themselves aprons.

> And they heard the voice of the LORD God walking in the garden in
> the cool of the day: and Adam and his wife hid themselves from the
> presence of the LORD God amongst the trees of the garden.
> And the LORD God called unto Adam, and said unto
> him, Where art thou?
> And he said, I heard thy voice in the garden, and I was afraid,
> because I was naked; and I hid myself.

God is understandably upset. He'd told them not to eat the fruit, after all, so he delivers a series of curses. For Eve, God punishes her with millennia of subservience to the male sex: "thy desire shall be to thy husband, and he shall rule over thee." For Adam, God damns him to an eternity of farming and baking: "thou shalt eat the herb of the field," God says, "In the sweat of thy face shalt thou eat bread."

Despite the bitter prognostications of God, however, Adam and Even continue to live together and get to the business of begetting—producing two sons, Cain and Abel. The Bible tells us all we need to know about how things are shaping up for the tribes of Israel: "And Abel was a keeper of sheep, but Cain was a tiller of the ground." This represents the first moment in the Bible of career choice— either head out to the fields to till and toil, or raise some cantankerous goats and sheep and get milking. Those are the only choices for the sons of Adam and Eve.

There are a multitude of interpretations of the story of Adam and Eve. From Talmudic studies to modern religious scholarship, the way in which scholars have analyzed the story is multifaceted. But what it is interesting is that Adam and Eve are outdoors, in a "state of nature" in a way that resembles outdoor experiences. This is important: within the Judeo-Christian construct, the very rules of God are put into play to restrict Adam and Eve's access to the outdoors. Left to their own devices, the outdoors serves to open up the avenue for evil and sin. This ideology is embedded in much of the efforts of the western world to colonize other peoples and develop industry.

What's interesting about this dynamic—the dark woods being full of evil that must be overcome—is that it's also responsible for so much of our moral framework in the west. The Judeo-Christian construct is actually necessary to provide a place for risk—an opportunity for growth. Stories with a strong Christian thread often play on the idea of overcoming the fear and challenges of nature—Dante begins his exploration in the *Inferno* by being "lost" in a dark wood. The idea of the wild as a place of challenge and obstacle is hardwired into stories. Venturing into the unknown is a necessary approach to growth. So the outdoors exists in this fascinating duality—a place that is both compelling and symbolic of some eternally lost ideal but also remains scary and risky.

Within education and in terms of the history of educational institutions, which are structured in large part on the religious education of the preceding centuries in Europe, this dynamic has served to make school fall under the purview of indoor, hierarchical structures rather than outdoor, collaborative ones. Outdoors equals sin; the intervention of divine justice has us turning the Garden of Eden into a sheep pasture. But the anti-outdoor philosophies of the developing world over the past few hundreds of years have gone even further—now even outdoor work is seen in some places as a humiliating experience to be avoided.

THE ESCAPE OF HUCK FINN

The prevailing prejudice against outdoor work—and outdoor learning—can be seen in the manner in which, even today, lighter skin is considered a symbol of the upper class; in some Asian cultures middle-class women try not to let their skin brown in the sun as it's considered a sign of peasantry. Browned skin means working outdoors, in the sun, whereas lighter tones symbolize an indoor life of leisure. For as long as humans have lived within a system where there were farmers who worked the land and a ruling class that owned it, maintaining distinctions between labor and owner have been hardwired into how to think about the inside, versus the outside world.

When we live in an indoor world, what are the most highly valued skills that can be taught? Numeracy, literacy, and citizenship are arguably—outside of religious instruction—three of the most consistent disciplines in the history of learning. And why shouldn't they be?

In early Mesopotamia, where the epic of Gilgamesh and Enkidu comes from, writing was created about 10,000 years ago, and scribes were initially responsible for taking stock (counting) of the worldly possessions of royalty or landowners. The amount of livestock, or quantity of grain. Scribes wrote bills of sale, kept ledgers. As for citizenry, they wrote laws, policies— recorded the decrees of kings. It was imperative that the individuals responsible for transcribing the words of the elite were supervised and controlled, lest they purposefully manipulate language in a way that could be negative for the ruling elite.

Even the story of Gilgamesh, arguably, is written to shore up the belief system of the ruling elite, with Gilgamesh—an urban king—as the hero. Later on, writing is used as a powerful tool to subvert the ruling elite—one thinks of the subversive effect of books like *Catcher in the Rye* had on American youth; Edward Abbey's *Monkey House Gang* had on the environmental movement of the latter twentieth century, or the way Martin Luther King Jr's "Letter from a Birmingham Jail" helped fan the flames of the civil rights movement.

These discriminatory systems of belief have led up to the present, when wild and ungovernable boys are deemed 'problems' because they don't submit to imposed order, and girls who play out in the dirt are seen as less "ladylike." What state-mandated education has always wanted from students is docility and obedience. The surest way to achieve this is by sticking children indoors, imprisoning them. Let them outside, and they could easily escape attempts to "civilize" them and light out for the territories like Huck Finn.

The reality is that the skills best suited for success in indoor schools are conscientious obedience to authority; those students who follow rules are generally rewarded with more awards and praise, thus accessing a greater share of opportunities. Before he can become Gilgamesh's boon companion, Enkidu must be shaved and civilized—brought down a peg from his beastly origins.

Another insidious scheme that exists within the structure of modern indoor schooling is the encouragement of intra-student competition. Like the movie *Hunger Games*, which pits various children against each other in gladiatorial combat so that their respective homelands will stay divided rather than band together against the fascist dictatorship, schools ensure that students won't resist by imposing a meritocracy in which those who are raised with material advantages perform better. Schools also award power to those most conditioned to sedentary passivity, thus the least likely to incite radical change in the system. Inherent in the structure of schools is that children are not autonomous. Being outdoors reinforces a sense of independence—it does not dovetail with the requirements of educational systems designed to enforce regulation and hegemony.

What the outdoors can engender in children is radical autonomy, self-reliance, and a willingness to participate in egalitarian systems of decision making. Schools don't make citizens; they make captives, doomed to repeat the very ideologies that denied people liberty in the first place.

Culturally, as a result of millennia of anti-nature propaganda on behalf of landowners and rulers like Gilgamesh (who may have been a real ruler, fictionalized in the poem), the Judeo-Christian tradition, and the ruling elite, it is traditional to revile outdoor creatures. The racially charged anti-indigenous movements of the eighteenth and nineteenth centuries in the United States and Australia were founded on the notion that the outdoor-living native populations were backward and subhuman—a designation we've held onto.

LEARNING TO BE SAVAGE

John Bodley is a cultural anthropology professor from the University of Washington. Bodley's work has in part focused on the way "progress"—defined as the introduction of traditional western notions of development, infrastructure, wealth, education, and health care—has affected indigenous populations around the world.

In his book *Victims of Progress*, Bodley tells the story of how the ethnocentric views of researchers in the mid-twentieth century established the theoretical counterpart to the systematic plundering of the developing world by established industrial nations. He offers an anecdote of Lord Fitzroy Raglan, who was the president of the Royal Anthropological Institute in Britain. Referring to the belief of tribal people the world over, he stated, "We should bring to them our justice, our education, and our science. Few will deny that these are better than anything which savages have got."

Forcing "civilization" down the throats of indigenous people was, really, its own industry during much of the nineteenth and twentieth centuries. The key word in the aforementioned quote by Lord Fitzroy Raglan is "education." The education in question—British schooling—was based on a pedagogy introduced during the industrial revolution. Sit the students, in rows, indoors, and get them to learn their ABCs. Dress them up like little Lord Fauntleroys, and deny them the exciting experience of living through the world around them, as tribal and indigenous people did.

Bodley's work deals with the way in which indigenous peoples have suffered at the hands of colonial powers eager to extract the resources contained in their homelands. The underlying argument used throughout history when a more technologically advanced culture invades and extracts the resources of a less technologically advanced peoples is that outdoor, small-scale, autonomous living was dirty, unproductive, and "backward." This discriminatory idea is so deeply hardwired into western thought that homelessness is seen as an affliction, and often equated to an epidemic or scourge—personal property and privacy reign supreme—and has carried over into multiple facets of culture.

Culturally, the idea that outdoor spaces that are left untenanted and wild are useless abound. When we speak of ideas we haven't turned into something productive or pragmatic, we say they are "fallow." Both "culture" and "cultivate" come from the same etymological root, suggesting that the very notion of culture involves chopping up the earth, planting rows of crops, and getting things in order. A more autonomous, foraging existence is outside of culture. For a long time, and even into the twentieth century, culture was synonymous with the kind of technological and bureaucratic structures that defined western Europe and America.

I called Bodley to get his take on outdoor education, to see if he thought that it might suffer from some of the same discrimination that indigenous peoples have experienced. After all, the similarities are striking. When you're out and about rambling through the woods, you're not really *doing* anything.

You move from place to place, set up camp, and hang out. Eat food. Get dirty. The outdoors has a tendency to erode traditional hierarchies and create more flexible, egalitarian social dynamics. There's plenty of time for lying about and catching a nap on a boulder in the sun. You don't really build anything since you can't carry much. Plans are loosely adhered to, as weather, health, and the strength of the group ebbs and flows and must be accounted for. Hardly the Victorian notion of agitated, industrious progress.

Bodley explained that an important thing to understand is that one of the essential components of the introduction of western ideas into indigenous settings has always been an increase in the scale of complexity. This is deemed as progress, naturally, and is a concept that we've adopted in education.

Trigonometry is seen as more "advanced" than finger painting because you've got to know all kinds of stuff to do it. To finger paint you just need fingers and paint. However, a finger-painter has all they need for their craft, whereas to practice trigonometry, one has to progress through school, have money to purchase books, have transportation to large buildings called schools that need heating and electricity, and whatnot. To learn trigonometry is to participate in ramping up the scale of complexity in multiple ways.

What happens when you increase the scale of complexity—for instance, replacing a fluid, loosely held system of animist beliefs shared by all in a tribe with the highly codified strictures of Catholicism that require the translation powers of a priest—is that you end up introducing dizzying levels of complicated hierarchy. And, of course, there is always a profit to be made. "There are people who benefit directly from increasing scales of complexity," Bodley told me. In the previous example, for instance, the Catholic Church has profited a great deal through the active and immensely successful proselytizing of their religion to indigenous peoples worldwide. Currently, they own about 177 million acres of land (plus Vatican City), ranking them third in the world for land ownership, squeezed out by King Abdullah from Saudi Arabia and the Queen of England.

In outdoor education, no one benefits disproportionately. Even instructors at organizations like Outward Bound and the National Outdoor Leadership School earn a pittance compared to the teachers and administration at most high schools. The reality is that schools mimic the very usurpation of independence and freedom that colonization and the industrial extraction of resources have around the globe.

Social stigma is now a powerful deterrent to outdoor living. People are considered "homeless" or "tramps" if they live outside. The only acceptable way to go about outdoor living is to insulate oneself with the badges of material wealth in the form of Patagonia fleece and North Face nylon—symbolic messages that while you may be spending time outside, you are securely ensconced in the material, civilized, indoor world. In fact, the only way to be "properly" outside is to be "inside" the right clothes.

The same is true for children. Those who play sports like football and baseball, with their rules and hierarchies and institution-reinforcing structures, are more likely to be seen as viable citizens than a kid who rambles through the fields all day after school. Princeton doesn't care if your kid can navigate the natural world in an authentic way. But if they can play defensive end, they'll take them. In fact, the uniforms of organized sports are, in a way, very real military-like signifiers of validity and loyalty—they erase identity, suggesting acquiescence to the goals of the team.

DRESS FOR SUCCESS

In fact, the modern workplace—and by extension schools—has inculcated this indoor ethos in the way we dress. Ceremonial dress has always played a role in human culture. Whether it's a feathered headdress or a tuxedo we have, as a species, identified important cultural rituals through ceremonial dress. This is true on many college campuses. Students put on ties for job fairs and visits to prospective employers to demonstrate that they can play the game—a symbolic demonstration that they are able to participate in the commercially oriented activities of the workplace.

Although most young children dress comfortably, they have a tendency to stop dressing—and moving—more and more as they progress through junior high and high school. And elementary-age students, while they may dress comfortably, are surrounded by adults who don't. Teachers and administrators alike dress in "business casual," sending the message that to be taken seriously, you must dress in indoor clothes that restrict movement and inhibit play and exploration.

There is nothing more movement inhibiting than the dominance of "business casual."

But there's a deeper issue here, one relevant to the academy and to teachers in high school on down to kindergarten. Clothing often denotes rank and role, and by adopting indoor dress, teachers corner themselves and reduce the opportunity for outdoor experience. There's been a pervasive, steady movement toward turning teachers into middle managers. This shift is apparent in the way public school teachers have been robbed of vital autonomy in the classroom and turned into meritocratic bean counters, whose main job is to scurry about trying to satisfy vacuous standards rather than teach purely and authentically from their own experience, passion, and intellect. "The clothes make the man" is a truism, and suggestive of the negation of personal expression in favor of an indoor uniform.

Socrates wore the simple robes of a philosopher—the idea being that anyone caught up in the confines of material artifice couldn't be pure in thought. The tradition has some pretty solid precedents—Jesus, Mohammed, the Buddha—all chose simple, functional garb to visually renounce both the dominant culture's adherence to hierarchies and material wealth and the commonly held attitudes toward the lower classes.

Monks, Gandhi, teachers, or radical leaders who are serious about their mission and their message often adopt a "costume" that sends a clear message: *I am not part of the ruling elite. What I offer is different and outside the reach of institutional decorum.* It is not just public school teachers who are being treated like middle managers. College professors more and more are given tasks and expectations more in line with managers than teachers and thinkers.

In order to offer real learning experiences for our students, it's important to send the right message. It should be clear that teachers stand apart from the machinations of government, religion, and commerce. Being outdoors, and introducing outdoor experiences as a central part of the daily activities of both children and teachers, allow for this new identity to develop.

If teachers are truly expected to illuminate young minds (and while it could sound like hyperbole and waxing poetic, from John Dewey to Sir Ken Robinson, the role of the teacher as an ideal has always been so), then it is essential that they occupy a space delineated from the churn of daily life. To a certain degree, teachers must be ascetics, focused on learning and improving the outer learning experiences, and inner worlds, of children.

TALK DIRTY TO ME

If teachers are to introduce outdoor education as a central tenet of education, they're going to have to go outside. They're going to get dirty.

The bias against the outdoors—and by extension outdoor learning—is as old as dirt. Literally. The outdoors—be it wilderness, back yard, or farm and field—is traditionally associated with dirt and grime and dust. This type of matter is associated with disease, illness, and germs. It's why your mother told you to wash your hands before dinner. But the same stuff is also associated with activities that are considered "lower" (farm work, manual labor—the stuff of peasants) than more refined activities. As a result of that thinking, westerners have traditionally associated dirty skin with dirty minds—even dirty souls. Again, in the quirkily brilliant book *Dust*, scholar Joseph Amato unearths the thinking behind this prejudice against soil and grit:

> Dust and dirt were traditionally associated with transgressors and transgressions. To be dirty, or grovel in the dirt, connoted indecency and immorality. Steering

clear of dust and dirt sustained the cultural order, affirmed moral rectitude, and, most important, assured those who were clean that they were also morally pure.

Though more difficult to identify, culturally the same prohibition against outdoor play is still present. It is not unusual to equate the refinements of indoor life with achievements of intellect. The muddy rural kid, smashing around the fields, is seen in a different light than the bespectacled, backpack laden suburban student slouching gracelessly to after-school tutors.

The very word used by western, colonial powers to denigrate indigenous peoples—"native"—is now used to empower a generation of smartphone-addicted teens. "Digital natives" are seen as the harbingers of a new world, where social and professional currency are measured in how well one navigates the internet—or how well one can converse in the rapidly evolving digi-speak of the web. Inclusion in this exclusive club relies on a passive disregard for historical context, and an enabling of a new techno-industrial complex that favors the wealthy and leaves the have-nots struggling in the wake of the broad-banded and well-equipped first world. This reversal of the idea of being "native" is at the core of the way colonialism and imperialism operate. It is through co-opting the customs of those to be subjugated that subjugation is so easily achieved.

The very stuff of being outdoors—dirt, mud, and real contact with the environment—is eschewed in favor of clean technologies and learning structures that are not resistant to a bit of rain and weather. This dominance of the indoors—and relegation of the outdoors to a lesser, more primal state—underpins much of contemporary educations bias against natural, outdoor, unstructured play. But just as the phrase "native" has been appropriated and repurposed by the tech circles, the very act of engaging with nature has been replaced by a virtual experience.

PIXELATED NATURE

Interestingly, being outdoors for long periods of time erodes the dominance of the new technocracy. The very symbol of modern intelligentsia—the sleek tablet with graceful fingers swiping and tapping their way across the screen—cannot survive a bit of rain. The further out into the natural world we go, the less influence—and relevance—our iPhones and screens have. Their batteries only last so long, and eventually they aren't even useful to chop kindling or dig holes. They truly are, in a physical, practical sense, useless.

It is an industry of profound size that we have created to exist in this indoor, learned state. Ergonomic chairs, ergonomic keyboards, ergonomic computer mouse. Desks, lamps, desk-lamps; a dizzying array of paperclip/

pen/Post-it note holders. We buy cell phones encased in plastic and metal and then buy cases of plastic and metal to put them in. Laptop computers are portable. They require plastic and foam and nylon carrying cases and turn every space into work space. They make anytime screen time.

To avoid the physical deformities that may result from reading an iPad flat on a table, we create and buy little faux-suede folders that double as little stands to angle our tablets just so. Some students come to school with over a thousand dollars of technology in their possession, yet they struggle to read a sentence. Technology is an industry built on the notion that learning happens, and happens best, only when confined to a room, out of the elements.

In the adult professional world, it may be worse. Professional acumen is measured by the technology each person carefully arranges in front of them in the meeting—each one setting up a command center of smartphones, laptops, and tablets to maximize the wired-ness and demonstrate their digital relevance. Meanwhile, these same people blink in the bright sunlight of day, stumbling about over the uneven turf of the world, lost when not tethered to their devices.

The fact is, defenders of the supposed egalitarianism of the internet can be found keening sharply whenever it is criticized, defending connectivity with the same erudition used to prop up free trade, globalism, and, 100 years ago, colonization. This rationale is behind every Apple ad you've ever seen.

In the western world, arguably the largest barrier to getting kids to spend more time outside is screen-based entertainment. The immediate gratification of video games is so powerful that kids can't resist their siren songs. Not only that, but we've taken the outdoor's natural adventure-producing geography and recreated it indoors. Video games have avatars leaping across rivers and swinging on vines, replicating the adventurous play that kids used to engage in without the help of binary code. As Rebecca Onion points out in a recent article in *The Atlantic*, even the nasty stuff kids used to play with in the form of goopy gunk, or more accurately, slime, has been co-opted by the commodified, adult world. Green Slime, the ubiquitous stuff that gets sploshed all over people on the Nickelodeon kids cable network, sold in toys stores, and is supposed to represent gross, adult-free "kid culture" has been used to create a commercially viable, parentally approved version of the muck and slime and stuff of outdoor play. Onion writes:

> It can't be a coincidence that, during the same decades that saw the ascendancy of green slime, kids have enjoyed fewer and fewer opportunities to go outdoors and play by themselves. Chances to mess around in the world without adult supervision have dwindled. Green slime—As Seen on TV or mixed up by Mom—takes the place of mud pies, pond algae, and the guts of that bird that's been moldering by the neighbor's fence for a few weeks. If green slime had a tagline, it'd be Gross™, for Indoor Kids.

The real outdoors doesn't actually work that way. It isn't packaged, or sold to children; it doesn't wash off easily nor does it provide immediate gratification. The outdoors is a complicated place, full of fun, certainly, but also full of discomfort and decision making. It requires navigation, interpretation, and processing. Being outdoors is both a simple thing to achieve and unimaginably complex to experience.

Some of the times I've been outdoors have been grounded in that complexity, particularly as a young man intent on "lighting out" for the territories. An example: when I was in high school, I decided to get out "on the road" and experience the world firsthand. It wasn't a particularly well-thought-out plan. My friend and I decided—for complicated reasons grounded in the sheer absence of rational thinking that defines the adolescent's worldview—to drop out of high school, hitch hike across America, and run away to California, where we'd start a rock band and live a life of hedonistic celebrity. We left notes for our parents and hitchhiked through New York State, heading west.

Our first night "sleeping rough" was in the boondocks of the Adirondacks, in the woods next to train tracks. We were terrified, and while the only things we experienced were lumbering raccoons and the exhilarating and sleep-disrupting shriek of a freight train rumbling by us twenty feet away, it was a formative experience that made a bed and a breakfast table look tantalizing.

It was a brief adventure—we'd come crawling back home, tails between our legs, in less than a week—but for me it highlighted the difficulty of living without running water, electricity, and all the conveniences of the modern world.

Being homeless has long been a symbol of destitution. Heroes of childhood imagination—Huck Finn, Frodo, even modern protagonists like Hugo from the eponymous novel who squats in a Paris train station—are all, in a sense, homeless. Kids or adults who choose (or are forced by dint of circumstance) to wander the open world are seen as social problems that require institutionalized response. They are seen as misfits, non-utilitarian figures who require the same attention as someone who is sick or mentally ill (sadly, there is a substantial portion of homeless people who are in fact mentally ill, some 15 percent, according to an article in the *Washington* Post titled "Five Myths About America's Homeless" from 2010).

One of the things I discovered in my brief time "tramping" was just how difficult private property is as a concept when you don't own any. America is a highly delineated space. Even state parks sometimes require a fee to sleep there. In Sweden, as in other Nordic countries, there is actually a law that protects the rights of those sleeping on the land: *allemansrätten,* literally "every man's right." But in negotiating land that is either private or public, tramping around requires a deep sense of propriety, weighing of consequences, and thought.

The games that children play that try and recreate the adventure of being outside or exploring old cellar holes and the forest swipe away all the consequences and risks that make going outside the vitiating experience it is—that make it the learning experience it is. Technology cannot replace the very real, and important, physical risks that accompany time spent outdoors for children. This is especially true for kids.

THE OUTDOOR GEOGRAPHY OF IMAGINATION

The growth of suburban neighborhoods has changed the way kids move through landscapes. It is not merely the prevalence and inexpensiveness of digital entertainment that keeps children indoors; it is the fact that the outdoors has ceased to be a place that they feel they can inhabit with relative freedom.

While there are some enviable neighborhoods where children cross each other's backyard and explore the bushy and sodden nooks of their territories regardless of who owns it, most modern neighborhoods have a very private, closed-off feel. Those who grew up during the mid- or latter part of the twentieth century in more rural or small town environments spent at least part of their free time tramping around the woods, field, and along the stream that ran behind homes. Never did concepts such as trespassing or property lines enter barmy childhood imagination. Woods, fields, and neglected corners of the world were under the ownership of kids by default.

The indoor world is intractably adult, while the outdoors used to represent the freedom of childhood, the release of the structures that the rule-dominated, adult-monitored spaces indoors represented. Now, with auto-centric urban planning, private property, stranger danger, kids with overscheduled lives, and of course the cocooning influence of digital technology, children's lives are crisscrossed with barriers that are practically insurmountable. How are they to gain access to their original frontier? They can't; it's gone.

In 1890, the U.S. Census reported that human density had reached a point that there was no longer any viable "frontier." Frederick Jackson Turner, a young historian, helped solidify this notion at the time. The irony, of course, is that the land had always been filled with people. Native Americans had settled and lived in every corner of the continent. What the white settlers of the North American Continent saw as empty land was empty because of the genocide inflicted on the Native American population over the preceding 300 years.

It's a remarkable analogy; just as we've settled into our digitally mediated, helicopter-parenting existence, the frontier of children's imagination has also closed. Once populated by kids dashing through yards and fields, exploring vacant lots, and claiming ownership of all the land and free spaces in between homes, now the vast stretches of suburban landscape are devoid of kids and their very symbolic meaning—free, unfettered by the restraints and responsibilities of the indoor world. To add another layer of complexity to the social conditions making outdoor time rarer for children is the way in which race plays a role. While getting outdoors for a suburban kid with an iPad and Xbox is tough, it is even more challenging for children from minority groups.

RACIAL ENVIRONMENTS

One of the greatest barriers to getting outdoors isn't mosquitoes or not having the right kind of hiking boots, but the color of your skin. According to a 2015 *New York Times* article by Glenn Nelson titled "Why Are Our Parks So White?" 37 percent of the population are people of color, but only 22 percent of visitors to National Parks are. Personal experience bears this out. Trekking in the Rockies, Sierras, or Green Mountains, the folks you're most likely to meet on the trail are white.

The construct is further realized in schools, where white, affluent kids are usually the ones going on school-sponsored outdoor excursions, visiting nature centers, and having outdoor experiences. The barrier between the outdoors and an African American child just don't exist for many middle- and upper-class white children.

Identifying the cause of barriers to the outdoors and assessing their impact on learning is essential if any real work is to be done in education toward imbuing the experience of intellectual and personal growth with the vital experiences to be had in the natural world. Compounding that is that the U.S. Census Bureau predicts an increase in the percentage of people of color in the U.S. population. In fact, by midcentury it's likely that the majority of U.S. citizens will be non-white.

Creating an educational system that values and implements programs that connect kids with nature is seen as one of the only ways to protect and manage our rapidly disappearing wildlands. If students of color are being denied those experiences, that's a massive swath of the population that will grow up without a personal connection to the outdoors, and without a deeply held conviction to protect its remaining undeveloped nooks and crannies.

Why don't African Americans, for example, go out hiking more? It's a question that's received a fair amount of attention, and one of the arguments often made is that the African American population is predominantly urban, therefore unlikely to take part in outdoor activities. Within this argument are two fallacies: one, that African Americans think differently about nature somehow, and two, that urban people don't access the outdoors through visiting national parks and undeveloped, natural terrain. The latter doesn't hold water: over 80 percent of the country is urban. Urban, suburban, and rural people and families visit the outdoors, whether national parks, state parks, or local nature preserves. The first assumption—that African Americans think differently about nature—is intensely problematic and possibly demonstrates an inherent racism. It's untrue.

African Americans (and other minorities) do in fact have a deep relationship with the outdoors. The obstacles that exist don't come from some internal bias within the African American community. In fact, that line of thinking—that black people are holding themselves back from some kind of outdoor experience due to some culturally specific set of ideas about nature— is thinking that shares much in common with some racist ideologies of the past. It puts the blame, or fault, for the statistical anomaly of less black people experiencing the outdoors per capita than white on the African American community, rather than identifying systematic ways in which certain populations have been denied access to various experiences through history.

Rashad Shabazz is an associate professor at the School of Social Transformation at Arizona State University. When he taught previously at UVM, we would often get our kids together and talk shop about teaching, research, and writing. Shabazz's work centers on the geography of race. He writes about the way the urban landscape plays a role in shaping people's understanding of racial identity. His book *Spatializing Blackness* focuses on the manner in which urban geography affects identity for young black men in Chicago.

I asked Shabazz about why he thought black people didn't seem to get out into nature as much as whites, according to statistics. Through his work, Shabazz has come to understand why people live where they do, what forces are at play that settle African Americans in cities and elsewhere, and why particular neighborhoods have a majority population of minorities. But in addition, he explores what constraints limit movement and relocation—what barriers exist for African Americans that limit their transition from one place to the next.

Getting outdoors, into nature, and engaging with a wild, unstructured environment requires only one thing, really. And that one thing has been systematically denied to African American communities through what Shabazz calls "historical patterns of segregation." The fact is, to set out and experience the woods, you've got to be able to get there. You've got to have *mobility*.

"Whiteness is associated with mobility, in the way that being male is associated with mobility," Shabazz said. This lack of mobility for communities of color—in particular African Americans—is real and concrete if you think of the ways cities have architectural infrastructures that box in ethnic neighborhoods with freeways, or the way access through public transportation as a pedestrian can be limited when traveling from an ethnic neighborhood to a downtown retail area, for instance. But this lack of mobility also exists on a less tangible level. The voyage required for an African American family to leave their neighborhood and head up into the mountains is one a white family—who may be used to gaining de facto access to both institutions and places for so long that it no longer even occurs to them—can't grasp.

This lack of mobility exists for students of color attending urban schools as well. While the specter of the "bias of low expectations" haunts schools filled mostly with African American or Latino kids, the real damage comes in how communities and governments respond to the challenges faced by these schools. The usual method is to put the pressure on and demand higher scores on standardized tests. The means by which this is achieved are usually by threatening the school with closure, or docking the pay of teachers or making funding contingent on acceptable scores. Panicked teachers respond the only way they can—by forcing their students to work harder, indoors, for longer and longer periods of time, further limiting their opportunity to experience the outdoors in any authentic way.

I know this from experience. When I worked at an urban charter school in Los Angeles, our funding (which came from the county) was dependent in part on how well we did on standardized tests. I blasted my middle schoolers with weeks of intense study to ensure that it wasn't my kids that lost us our charter. They resented it, I resented it, and I'm not sure how much learning—if any—actually took place.

There's an "inherent institutional bias towards providing different educational experiences" for white kids and black kids, Shabazz pointed out, and the failure to get students of color out and about in nature is one of the way it manifests itself.

If we're going to talk about how to improve education—either through getting students outdoors more or through some other means—we have to address the glaring reality that students of color don't have the same experience as white students. The system they are faced with is one rooted in a historical continuum informed by racist policies of the past.

A larger cultural narrative is at work here, one in which the way we relate to nature is different depending on the color of our skin. In his book *Race and Nature*, author Paul Outka states:

> This legacy—in which whites viewed black people as part of the natural world, and then proceeded to treat them with same mixture of contempt, false reverence, and real exploitation that also marks American environmental history— inevitably makes the possibility of an *uncomplicated* union with the natural world less readily available to African Americans than it has been to whites, who, by and large, have not suffered from such a history.

The way in which we think about ourselves in relation to nature is defined in part with how and where we were raised, but also by large-scale, sweeping historical narratives that inform our broad understanding of our place in society. "The dominant environmental narrative in the United States is primarily constructed and informed by white, western European, or EuroAmerican voices," writes Carolyn Finney in *Black Faces, White Spaces*, her book on the hidden history of African American environmentalism.

In fact, as Finney points out, there is a robust history of African American environmentalists. But the outdoors is seen within contemporary society through the lens of media and advertising, and, more and more, through social media. When the internet spews forth images of families exploring nature, they are almost always white and wealthy. While there are a few exceptions, the overwhelming influence of this social construction is just yet another barrier for people of color to explore the outdoors. Education plays an outsized role in the opportunities that exist to correct this—the question remains how schools should approach getting children—all children, regardless of race—outdoors more to capitalize on the benefits.

A SCHOOL WITHOUT WALLS

What would an outdoor school look like? How would it function? These and other similar questions face educators who see the value of rugged, outdoor experiences for children. There's no single answer, but instead a collage of intersecting theories, realities, and practical steps that teachers and parents alike must unsnarl to start moving toward authentic outdoor learning experiences.

There are many places in the world where outdoor education sits firmly nested as a vital part of the curriculum—indeed, even the social fabric. Outdoor kindergartens in Germany, and a growing movement of outdoor schools for younger children across Europe, point to an increasing understanding of the need for just these types of learning environments.

Here in the States, schools from Washington to Vermont are beginning to push outdoor components as part of the education they offer. Just down the road from where I live in Vermont, there's a school called The Walden Project—an offshoot of a local public high school that teachers students outside, in the woods, every day. These programs are a vital and necessary step, but the risk is the same that faces art, music, and theater programs nationwide: if the program doesn't directly and obviously improved test scores (which is attached to funding for many institutions), then it's on the chopping block, despite that overwhelming evidence that they *do* in fact increase student learning across disciplines. Not only do educators and parents need to understand the philosophic, intellectual, physical, psychological, and cultural underpinnings of outdoor education; we need to make it a systemic part of our educational infrastructure.

You'd think a place like Finland—small, close to the Arctic, and tucked away from the hub of Europe way up near places like Latvia and Estonia—would be good for only reindeer burgers and frostbite. You'd be wrong. Finland has one of the highest standards of living in the world (in the top 25 according to the United Nations Human Development Index) and one of the highest-ranked educational systems globally according to various indexes and reports, including one by Pearson, an education firm. So if Finland is so great—what gives? And why is it that if you Google "Finland" and "education," you inevitably get articles galore about how students go outside no matter the temperature, and do so all the time?

Outdoor education—really, just time spent outdoors under the guidance of trained, invested adults—is a cultural cornerstone of Finnish education. In fact, outdoor education is positioned in such a way that it's tied directly to National Core Curriculums for both basic education and upper secondary schools. The Finnish National Board of Education has included outdoor learning as an integral part of their education, as fundamental as reading, writing, and arithmetic. In fact, in the National Core Curriculum for students aged seven to sixteen, the designers of Finnish education are explicit in their aims for outdoor education:

> To raise environmentally conscious citizens who are committed to a sustainable way of life. The schools must teach future-oriented thinking and building the future on ecologically, economically, socially, and culturally sustainable premises.

Before you go thinking that Finland is home to a bunch of elves and trolls knitting reindeer yarn hats and living in gingerbread houses, remember that it's home to Nokia, a technology company ranked within the top 300 largest companies in the world, and also a hotbed of new and developing technology start-ups according to *Forbes* magazine. It's an example of a country that sits firmly within a cultural tradition of exploring the outdoors as means of personal development without sacrificing participation in the modern world—two poles that often seem incompatible but aren't.

Not only are outdoor experiences—like fifteen minutes of outdoor play for every forty-five of classroom work—a central part of Finnish schools, but the doctrine and philosophy developed by the Finnish Board of Education directly references the importance of rigorous outdoor adventures. While not necessarily compulsory, it is so much a part of the cultural heritage that outdoor excursions and adventures are simply seen as part of the normal trajectory of a child's development.

One of the most fascinating aspects of how Finland approaches education is their understanding of the interdisciplinary way outdoor adventure educates students. The approach teachers take is one in which sensitivity, scientific observation, and ethics are considered—all within the realm of experiential education. And it's not just in the younger grades that outdoor learning is a key component. Even at university students are engaged with outdoor learning as a central part of their educational experience.

What Finland has done—and indeed, what is possible for American schools—is inculcate educational pedagogy with the cultural imperative to get *outside*. Treks in the forest and mountains are a simple rite of passage for young Scandinavians, and it is their unremarkableness that is so remarkable. Using schools to get children out experiencing nature allows them the opportunity to escape, if even for a brief time, the weight of institutionalized expectations and structures. It allows them time to breathe.

Gilgamesh is a hero, but also a king and politician, bent on securing his fame through great deeds. He drags Enkidu with him on all manner of exploits, killing monsters in the cedar forest and even ending up in the underworld. But one can't help but think that Enkidu, who lived a life outdoors free from the concerns of the city state, free from the imposition of institutionalized legacy, must've lamented the loss of his time in nature, free from the harried, exhausting life of civilization. Better, sometimes, to stay out at the water hole with the gazelles, watching the light flicker across the surface.

Conclusion

The Outdoor Nation Proclamation

There are a number of schools of thought—attributed to such individuals as Thomas Jefferson, Aristotle, John Dewey, and others—that go, in broad strokes, something like this: in order for democracy to work, we must have an educated citizenry. Now to be clear, I am not a political theorist, but that sounds like a pretty solid assumption to me. It seems self-evident that education should largely be concerned with increasing the individual student's capacity for personal and intellectual growth, but that it's not just the solipsistic exercise of making ourselves or our students smart for smartness sake. Rather, education should create scenarios in which educated people will—ideally—seek to spread that education to others. Lift others as they themselves have been lifted.

Again, I'm no political ideologue. But I would argue that freedom and liberty are at the core of what we do as educators. And I would extend that notion to parents. Those of us with children want free-thinking kids to grow up to be independent, strong, fulfilled individuals. We want our children to live lives that have *meaning*. Embracing those ideas of growth and development in our pedagogy, in our personal philosophies, in our parenting, and in our very own lives is essential to the work of teaching and raising children. Our job—if I may be so bold—is to imbue children with those ideals. To give them the empowering gift of free thinking, and the liberty to learn as much and for as long as they may.

A large part of that freedom is gained by releasing childhood from the demands of transactional education—breaking the bonds of social obligation driven by common-sense falsehoods and letting our children have a bit of free range to explore. The landscapes we inhabit in the real world are reflected in our own internal, ideological terrains. If we truly want education to offer unrestricted access to the world of ideas, we must give our children the absolute freedom to explore the outdoor world.

We are living in a world that is increasingly unfriendly to children. Autocentric urban planning, standards-based school curricula, digital entertainment that replaces active engagement with passive absorption, a culture of risk aversion, and the growing influence of job-skills related to educational models and schools driven by economic narratives rather than authentic learning. Our children and students dutifully shuffle from one benchmark to the next, wearily resigned to see school as a necessary confinement that diminishes their autonomy and rewards complacent acquiescence.

How to regain, then, the action-filled adventure of childhood? It's not as though we're wearing rose-tinted glasses looking back on some imaginary halcyon days. Many aspects of childhood are wonderfully improved: tolerance, inclusion, and celebration of diversity have made leaps and bounds over the past several decades. But there is much work to be done to give children back their childhood.

The pathway to this freedom leads outdoors.

The etymology of the word "freedom" is curious. "Free" is from the Middle English world *fre* or *freo*. Tracing it all the back through Old High German, we find the Gothic variation *freis*, which can be compared to the old Norse word *frithr*. It means love, or peace. This deeper historical meaning of the word "free" is interesting for a few reasons. Not only are "love" and "peace" at the heart of the word "freedom," but the words from which "freedom" is derived is closely related to another Old High German word, *friunt*, which means friend. At the heart of freedom is friendship.

What of the freedom to be found in the outdoors? What sort of freedom is it? Is it different from other forms of freedom? Many proponents of "freedom," particularly within the American political landscape, seem to feel that freedom is something to be defended; thus, it is something to be owned, since it can be stolen. Doesn't sound all that free, really.

In the relationship between the words "love" and "freedom" and "friend" we find a densely layered history of the concept of true freedom. We see that it is only in love—in friendship—that we can truly be free. And our first loves, our purest loves, are those we have for the world around us, and the people immediately in it. A friend or two, the trees, stars, and the wide open, uncrowded world.

If what we seek for our children and students is true freedom; freedom from bias and prejudice, freedom from dogmatism and ignorance—the kind of freedom that seeks to empower those in possession of freedom with the opportunity to give freedom to others—then that freedom comes from early and sustained contact with the wild world of nature.

Works Cited

Aamodt, Sandra, and Sam Wang. "The Sun Is the Best Optometrist." *The New York Times*. 20 June 2011. Web. 21 October 2015.

"About the OECD."—OECD. http://www.oecd.org/about/ N.p., n.d. Web. 16 September 2015.

Achebe, Chinua. *Things Fall Apart*. Broomall, PA: Chelsea House, 2002. Print.

Alexie, Sherman. *The Absolutely True Diary of a Part-Time Indian*. London: Andersen, 2015. Print.

Amato, Joseph A. *Dust: A History of the Small and the Invisible* University of California Press, 2000.

Ananthaswamy, Anil. "Why Is Exercise Such a Chore?" *Slate Magazine*. N.p., 16 June 2013. Web. 10 July 2017.

Andrews, Paul W., and J. Anderson Thompson, Jr. "Depression's Evolutionary Roots." *Scientific American*. N.p., 25 August 2009. Web.

Andrews, Paul W., and J. Anderson Thompson. "The Bright Side of Being Blue: Depression as an Adaptation for Analyzing Complex Problems." *Psychological Review* 116.3 (2009): 620–54. Web.

Baldwin, James. *Notes of a Native Son*. Ed. Edward P. Jones. Boston: Beacon, 2012. Print.

Barash, David P. "God, Darwin and My College Biology Class." *The New York Times*. 27 September 2014. Web. 7 June 2016.

Behn, Aphra, Catherine Gallagher, and Simon Stern. *Oroonoko, Or, The Royal Slave*. Boston: Bedford/St. Martin's, 2000. Print.

Berkowitz, Bonnie, and Patterson Clark. "The Health Hazards of Sitting." *The Washington Post*. WP Company, January 2014. Web. 10 July 2017.

Biba, Erin. "The Way the U.S. Teaches Science Doesn't Work." *Popular Science*. N.p., 5 September 2013. Web. 7 June 2016.

Birkerts, Sven. "Green Light." *Brevity A Journal of Concise Literary Nonfiction*. N.p., January 2013. Web. 5 October 2015.

Blum, Susan D. *"I Love Learning; I Hate School."* An Anthropology of College. Ithaca, NY: Cornell University Press, 2016. Print.

Bodley, John H. *Victims of Progress.* Menlo Park, CA: Cummings Publications, 1975. Print.

Bowler, Diana E., Lisette M. Buyung-Ali, Teri M. Knight, and Andrew S. Pullin. "A Systematic Review of Evidence for the Added Benefits to Health of Exposure to Natural Environments." *BMC Public Health* 10.1 (2010): 456. Web.

Bucholtz, Mary. "'Why Be Normal?': Language and Identity Practices in a Community of Nerd Girls." *Language in Society* 28 (1999): n. pag. Web.

Carey, Benedict. "Antidepressant Paxil Is Unsafe for Teenagers, New Analysis Says." *The New York Times.* 16 September 2015. Web. 18 December 2015.

Cervinka, R., K. Roderer, and E. Hefler. "Are Nature Lovers Happy? On Various Indicators of Well-Being and Connectedness with Nature." *Journal of Health Psychology* 17.3 (2011): 379–88. Web.

Chatwin, Bruce. *The Songlines.* New York: Penguin, 2012. Print.

"Climate Change Evidence: How Do We Know?" *Climate Change: Vital Signs of the Planet.* N.p., n.d. Web. 14 September 2015.

Cohen, Noam. "We're All Nerds Now." *The New York Times.* 13 September 2014. Web. 18 December 2015.

Coleman, Alison. "A New Generation of Tech Disruptors Is Thriving in Finland." *Forbes.* 30 October 2015. Web. 7 June 2016.

Coleman, Mark. "Why Meditating in Nature Is Easier | Outdoors Meditation for Beginners." *Yoga Journal.* 10 December 2014. Web. 16 January 2017.

Conrad, Joseph, and Paul B. Armstrong. *Heart of Darkness.* New York: W.W. Norton, 2017. Print.

Cook, M. I. "Effects of Short-Term Hunger and Competitive Asymmetry on Facultative Aggression in Nestling Black Guillemots Cepphus Grylle." *Behavioral Ecology* 11.3 (2000): 282–87. Web.

Culhane, Dennis. "Five Myths about America's Homeless." *Washington Post.* N.p., 11 July 2010. Web. 12 January 2016.

Defoe, Daniel. *Robinson Crusoe.* Ed. Michael Shinagel. New York: Norton, 1975. Print.

"Depression." Centers for Disease Control and Prevention, 17 July 2015. Web. 18 December 2015.

Dika, S. L., and K. Singh. "Applications of Social Capital in Educational Literature: A Critical Synthesis." *Review of Educational Research* 72.1 (2002): 31–60. Web.

Dillard, Annie. *Pilgrim at Tinker Creek; An American Childhood; The Writing Life.* New York: Quality Paperback Book Club, 1990. Print.

Dogan, Elie. "The Myopia Boom." *Nature.* Nature Publishing Group, 18 March 2015. Web. 21 October 2015.

Doughty, Del. "Inside Higher Ed." *A Professor Takes His Classes on a Walk (essay).* Inside Higher Ed., 31 May 2016. Web. 10 July 2017.

Dreifus, Claudia. "Ideas for Improving Science Education in the U.S." *The New York Times.* 2 September 2013. Web. 7 June 2016.

Drew, Christopher. "Why Science Majors Change Their Minds (It's Just So Darn Hard)." *The New York Times.* 5 November 2011. Web. 7 June 2016.

Eberle, Scott G. "The Elements of Play: Towards a Philosophy and a Definition of Play." *Journal of Play* 6.2 (2014): n. pag. Print.

"Education at a Glance 2014." *Education at a Glance* (2014): n.p. Organisation for Economic Co-operation and Development. Web.

Ellis, Frank H. *Twentieth Century Interpretations of Robinson Crusoe: A Collection of Critical Essays*. Englewood Cliffs, NJ: Prentice-Hall, 1969. Print.

Ellison, Ralph. *Invisible Man*. Bronx, NY: Ishi International, 2015. Print.

Eliot, George. *Daniel Deronda.* Penguin Books, 1995.

Eliot, George. Middlemarch. Penguin Books, 2003.

"Facts & Statistics | Anxiety and Depression Association of America, ADAA." *Facts & Statistics | Anxiety and Depression Association of America, ADAA*. N.p., n.d. Web. 6 January 2016.

Finney, Carolyn. *Black Faces, White Spaces: Reimagining the Relationship of African Americans to the Great Outdoors*. Chapel Hill: University of North Carolina, 2014. Print.

"5 Animals That Have Gone Extinct in the Past 50 Years." *PlanetSave*. N.p., 31 May 2015. Web. 14 September 2015.

Foster, Charles. *Being a Beast: Adventures across the Species Divide*. N.p.: PICADOR USA, 2017. Print.

Freire, Paulo. *Pedagogy of the Oppressed*. New York: Continuum, 2000. Print.

Gallagher, Emily. "Department of Applied Psychology." *The Effects of Teacher-Student Relationships: Social and Academic Outcomes of Low-Income Middle and High School Students—Applied Psychology OPUS—NYU Steinhardt*. NYU Steinhardt Department of Applied Psychology, n.d. Web. 16 January 2017.

Gardner, John Champlin. *On Moral Fiction*. New York: Basic, 1992. Print.

George, Jean Craighead. *Julie of the Wolves*. N.p.: HarperCollins Childrens Books, 2016. Print.

George, Jean Craighead. *My Side of the Mountain*. New York: Puffin, 2012. Print.

Gould, Stephen Jay. *The Flamingo's Smile: Reflections in Natural History*. New York: W.W. Norton, 1987. Print.

Gray, Peter. "The Decline of Play and Rise in Children's Mental Disorders." *Psychology Today*. N.p., 26 January 2010. Web. 18 December 2015.

Greenfield, Susan. *Mind Change How Digital Technologies Are Leaving Their Mark on Our Brains*. New York: Random House, 2015. Print.

Hamann, Johann Georg. Writings on Philosophy and Language. Edited by Kenneth Haynes, Cambridge University Press, 2007.

Harris, Michael. *The End of Absence: Reclaiming What We've Lost in a World of Constant Connection*. New York: Current, 2014. Print.

Henriques, Gregg. "What Is Mindfulness and How Does It Work?" *Psychology Today*. N.p., 6 February 2015. Web. 16 January 2017.

Hepler, Cassie. "Philly Free School Offers Public, Private School Alternative." *Philly Free School Offers Public, Private School Alternative | Philadelphia Public Record*. Philadelphia Public Record, 4 February 2016. Web. 16 January 2017.

Hidaka, Brandon H. "Depression as a Disease of Modernity: Explanations for Increasing Prevalence." *Journal of Affective Disorders* 140.3 (2012): 205–14. Web.

Holmes, Joshua. "Building Bridges and Breaking Boundaries: Modernity and Agoraphobia." *Opticon 1826* (2006): n. pag. 2006. Web.

"Home | Pearson | The Learning Curve." http://thelearningcurve.pearson.com/ *Home | Pearson | The Learning Curve*. N.p., n.d. Web. 7 June 2016.

"How Many Species Are We Losing?" www.wwf.panda.org. N.p., n.d. Web. 14 September 2015.

Hughes, Jan, and Oi-Man Kwok. "Influence of Student-Teacher and Parent-Teacher Relationships on Lower Achieving Readers' Engagement and Achievement in the Primary Grades." *Journal of Educational Psychology* 99.1 (2007): 39–51. Web.

Hughes, Jan N., Wen Luo, Oi-Man Kwok, and Linda K. Loyd. "Teacher-Student Support, Effortful Engagement, and Achievement: A 3-Year Longitudinal Study." *Journal of Educational Psychology* 100.1 (2008): 1–14. Web.

"Human Development Reports." *Human Development Index (HDI)*. N.p., n.d. Web. 7 June 2016.

Hunt, Jasper S. *Ethical Issues in Experiential Education*. Dubuque, IA: Kendall/Hunt Pub., 1994. Print.

Ibsen, Henrik, and John R. Northam. *Ibsen's Poems*. Oslo: Norwegian University Press, 1986. Print.

Illich, Ivan. *Deschooling Society*. New York: Harper & Row, 1971. Print.

"IUCN, the International Union for Conservation of Nature." IUCN. N.p., n.d. Web. 14 September 2015.

John, Oliver P., Richard W. Robins, and Lawrence A. Pervin. *Handbook of Personality: Theory and Research*. New York: Guilford, 2011. Print.

Johnson, James E., Scott G. Eberle, Thomas S. Henricks, and David Kuschner. *Handbook of the Study of Play*. Lanham, MD: Rowman & Littlefield., 2015. Print.

Jones, Gerard. *Killing Monsters: Why Children Need Fantasy, Super Heroes, and Make-Believe Violence*. New York: Basic, 2002. Print.

Jones, Helen. "Risks of Biodiversity Loss Pose a Global Threat." The Wall Street Journal. Dow Jones & Company, n.d. Web.

Kesling, Ben. "Technology in Classrooms Doesn't Always Boost Education Results, OECD Says." *WSJ*. N.p., 15 September 2015. Web. 9 June 2016.

Kierkegaard, Soren. Fear and Trembling. Translated by Alastair Hannay, Penguin Books, 2003.

Kincaid, Jamaica. *A Small Place*. New York: Farrar, Straus, Giroux, 2000. Print.

Kolata, Gina. "Brown Fat, Triggered by Cold or Exercise, May Yield a Key to Weight Control." *The New York Times*. 24 January 2012. Web. 5 January 2016.

Kruijshaar, Michelle Elisabeth, Jan Barendregt, Theo Vos, Ron De Graaf, Jan Spijker, and Gavin Andrews. "Lifetime Prevalence Estimates of Major Depression: An Indirect Estimation Method and a Quantification of Recall Bias." *Eur J Epidemiol European Journal of Epidemiology* 20.1 (2005): 103–11. Web.

Kurzban, Robert. "Angry (Hungry) Birds | Evolutionary Psychology Blog." *Angry (Hungry) Birds*. N.p., 15 April 2014. Web. 6 January 2016.

La Canna, Xavier. "Prince Harry 'May Need Binoculars' to Match 'Super Sight' of Indigenous Soldiers." *ABC News*. N.p., 8 April 2015. Web. 21 October 2015.

Lans, Anouk A.j.j. Van Der, Joris Hoeks, Boudewijn Brans, Guy H.e.j. Vijgen, Mariëlle G.w. Visser, Maarten J. Vosselman, Jan Hansen, Johanna A. Jörgensen,

Jun Wu, Felix M. Mottaghy, Patrick Schrauwen, and Wouter D. Van Marken Lichtenbelt. "Cold Acclimation Recruits Human Brown Fat and Increases Nonshivering Thermogenesis." *Journal of Clinical Investigation*. 123.8 (2013): 3395–403. Web.

"Learning Disabilities." *The State of Learning Disabilities* (n.d.): n. pag. The National Center for Learning Disabilities, 2014. Web.

Lichtenbelt, Wouter Van Marken, Boris Kingma, Anouk Van Der Lans, and Lisje Schellen. "Cold Exposure—An Approach to Increasing Energy Expenditure in Humans." *Trends in Endocrinology & Metabolism* 25.4 (2014): 165–67. Web.

Liebenberg, Louis. *The Art of Tracking: The Origin of Science*. Claremont, CA: David Philip, 2001. Print.

Lieberman, Daniel E., and Dennis M. Bramble. "The evolution of marathon running: Capabilities in humans." *Sports Medicine* 37.4–5 (2007): 288–290.

Louv, Richard. *Last Child in the Woods: Saving Our Children from Nature-Deficit Disorder*. London: Atlantic, 2010. Print.

McAdams, Dan P., and McLean, Kate A. "Narrative Identity" *Current Directions in Psychological Science* 22.3 (2013).

Mariotti, Shannon L. *Thoreau's Democratic Withdrawal: Alienation, Participation, and Modernity*. Madison, WI: U of Wisconsin, 2010. Print.

Mascarenhas, GlobalPost Hyacinth. "13 Species We Might Have to Say Goodbye to in 2015." *USA Today*. Gannett, 2 January 2015. Web. 16 September 2015.

Maslow, Abraham. *Toward a Psychology of Being*. New York: Wiley, 1998. Print.

Mattson, Mark P. "Superior Pattern Processing Is the Essence of the Evolved Human Brain." *Frontiers*. 5 August 2014. Web. 10 July 2017.

McEnery, Thornton. "The World's 15 Biggest Landowners." *Business Insider*. 18 March 2011. Web. 6 January 2016.

Mongeau, Lillian. "Preschool without Walls." *The New York Times*. 30 December 2015. Web. 12 January 2016.

Montaigne, Michel de. *The Complete Essays* translated by M. A. Screech, Penguin Books, 2003.

Morrison, C. M., and Helen Gore. "The Relationship between Excessive Internet Use and Depression: A Questionnaire-Based Study of 1,319 Young People and Adults." *Psychopathology* 43.2 (2010): 121–26. Web.

MPH, Elizabeth D. Kantor. "Prescription Drug Use in US Adults 1999–2012." *JAMA.*, 3 November 2015. Web. 10 July 2017.

Muir, John. *The Mountains of California*. Boston: Houghton Mifflin, 1917. Print.

Muir, John. *My First Summer in the Sierra*. N.p.: Kessinger Publications, 2000. Print.

Murray, Christopher. "Parent and Teacher Relationships as Predictors of School Engagement and Functioning among Low-Income Urban Youth." *The Journal of Early Adolescence* 29.3 (2009): 376–404. Web.

Neiwert, David A. *Of Orcas and Men: What Killer Whales Can Teach Us*. New York: Overlook, 2015. Print.

Nelson, Glenn. "Opinion | Why Are Our Parks So White?" *The New York Times*. 10 July 2015. Web. 10 July 2017.

Novotney, Amy. "Getting Back to the Great Outdoors." *American Psychological Association*. N.p., March 2008. Web. 16 January 2017.

Olfson, Mark, Steven C. Marcus, and Benjamin G. Druss. "Effects of Food and Drug Administration Warnings on Antidepressant Use in a National Sample." *Archives of General Psychiatry* 65.1 (2008): 94. Web.

Olfson, Mark, et al. "Treatment of Young People With Antipsychotic Medications in the United States." JAMA Psychiatry, 72.9 (2015).

Onion, Rebecca. "Ode to Green Slime." *The Atlantic.* 6 February 2015. Web. 9 June 2016.

"Outdoor Play Linked to Children's Mental Health." *The Sydney Morning Herald.* 7 October 2010. Web. 10 July 2017.

Outka, Paul. *Race and Nature from Transcendentalism to the Harlem Renaissance.* New York: Palgrave Macmillan, 2013. Print.

"Overweight and Obesity Statistics." *Overweight and Obesity Statistics.* N.p., n.d. Web. 5 January 2016.

Panksepp, Jaak. "Affective Neuroscience of the Emotional BrainMind: Evolutionary Perspectives and Implications for Understanding Depression." *Dialogues in Clinical Neuroscience.* December 2010. Web. 10 July 2017.

Partridge, Eric. *Origins: A Short Etymological Dictionary of Modern English.* The Macmillan Company, New York, 1958.

"People and Events: The Closing of the American Wilderness." *PBS*, n.d. Web. 9 June 2016.

Pfeifer, Gaby. "How Personal Is Personal Development?" *Psychology Today.* N.p., 14 August 2016. Web. 16 January 2017.

Proust, Marcel, Lydia Davis, and Christopher Prendergast. *Swann's Way.* New York: Viking, 2003. Print.

Reynolds, Gretchen. "How Walking in Nature Changes the Brain." *The New York Times.* 22 July 2015. Web. 18 December 2015.

Rickett, Arthur. *The Vagabond in Literature: With 6 Portr.* London: J. M. Dent, 1906. Print.

Rose, Kathryn A., Ian G. Morgan, Wayne Smith, George Burlutsky, Paul Mitchell, and Seang-Mei Saw. "Myopia, Lifestyle, and Schooling in Students of Chinese Ethnicity in Singapore and Sydney." *Archives of Ophthalmology,* 126.4 (2008): 527. Web.

Rotman, Michael. "Cuyahoga River Fire | Cleveland Historical." Clevelandhistorical. org. Center for Public History + Digital Humanities at Cleveland State University, n.d. Web. 15 March 2016.

Rousseau, Jean-Jacques. *Emile.* Trans. Barbara Foxley. London: Dent, 1974. Print.

Russell, George K., ed. *Children & Nature: Making Connections.* Great Barrington, MA: Myrin Institute, 2014. Print.

Russell, Kent. *I Am Sorry to Think I Have Raised a Timid Son: Essays.* New York: Random House, 2015. Print.

Ryan, Richard M., Netta Weinstein, Jessey Bernstein, Kirk Warren Brown, Louis Mistretta, and Marylène Gagné. "Vitalizing Effects of Being Outdoors and in Nature." *Journal of Environmental Psychology* 30.2 (2010): 159–68. Web.

Safina, Carl. *Beyond Words: What Animals Think and Feel.* New York: Henry Holt and, LLC, 2015. Print.

Salis, Amanda. "Feeling Hangry? Why We Can Get Grumpy When We're Hungry." *Independent UK*. N.p., 20 July 2015. Web.

Sammons, Matthew F., and David A. Price. "Modulation of Adipose Tissue Thermogenesis as a Method for Increasing Energy Expenditure." *Modulation of Adipose Tissue Thermogenesis as a Method for Increasing Energy Expenditure*. Bioorganic & Medicinal Chemistry Letters, 10 December 2013. Web. 5 January 2016.

Sanders, Scott Russell. "Book World Review: 'The Adventures of Henry Thoreau,' by Michael Sims." *Washington Post*. N.d. Web. 18 December 2015.

"Schools Wasting Money on Computers for Kids: OECD." CNBC. N.p., 15 September 2015. Web. 16 September 2015.

Shabazz, Rashad. *Spatializing Blackness Architectures of Confinement and Black Masculinity in Chicago*. Urbana: University of Illinois, 2015. Print.

Shelley, Mary. *Frankenstein* W.W. Norton and Company, New York 1996.

"Threats to Biodiversity and Ecosystems." *Threats to Biodiversity and Ecosystems*. N.p., n.d. Web. 14 September 2015.

Townsend, Kristy L. "Brown fat fuel utilization and thermogenesis" *Trends in Endocrinology & Metabolism* "http://www.cell.com/trends/endocrinology-metabolism/issue?pii=S1043-2760(14)X0004-4" 25.4, April 2014.

Townsend, Kristy L., and Yu-Hua Tseng. "Brown Fat Fuel Utilization and Thermogenesis." *Trends in Endocrinology & Metabolism* 25.4 (2014): 168–77. Web.

Twain, Mark. *Adventures of Huckleberry Finn*. Ed. Henry Nash Smith. Boston, MA: Houghton Mifflin, 1958. Print.

Waal, Frans De. *Are We Smart Enough to Know How Smart Animals Are?* s.l.: Granta, 2017. Print.

The Wall Street Journal. Dow Jones & Company, n.d. Web. 14 September 2015.

Walker, Tim. "How Finland Keeps Kids Focused through Free Play." *The Atlantic*. 30 June 2014. Web. 7 June 2016.

Watson, Paul J., and Paul W. Andrews. "Toward a Revised Evolutionary Adaptationist Analysis of Depression: The Social Navigation Hypothesis." *Journal of Affective Disorders* 72.1 (2002): 1–14. Web.

Weinstein, N., A. K. Przybylski, and R. M. Ryan. "Can Nature Make Us More Caring? Effects of Immersion in Nature on Intrinsic Aspirations and Generosity." *Personality and Social Psychology Bulletin* 35.10 (2009): 1315–329. Web.

Weinstein, Netta, Jessy Bernstein, Kirk Warren Brown, Louis Mastella, and Marylene Gagne. "Spending Time in Nature Makes People Feel More Alive, Study Shows." *Rochester News*. N.p., 3 June 2010. Web. 16 January 2017.

Weintraub, Pamela. "July/August 2017." *Discover Magazine*. N.p., 31 May 2012. Web. 10 July 2017.

Wells, H. G., Shirley Bogart, and Brendan Lynch. *The Time Machine*. New York: Baronet, 2008. Print.

"Why the Common Core Flunks on Civic Education." *Washington Post*. N.d. Web. 14 September 2015.

Wilson, Edward O. *Naturalist*. Washington, D.C.: Island/Shearwater, 2006. Print.

Woolf, Virginia. *The Common Reader: First Series*. Ed. Andrew McNeillie. San Diego, CA: Harcourt Brace Jovanovich, 1986. Print.

Wurdinger, Scott D. *Philosophical Issues in Adventure Education*. Dubuque, IA: Kendall/Hunt Pub., 1997. Print.

Yoneshiro, Takeshi, Sayuri Aita, Mami Matsushita, Takashi Kayahara, Toshimitsu Kameya, Yuko Kawai, Toshihiko Iwanaga, and Masayuki Saito. "Recruited Brown Adipose Tissue as an Antiobesity Agent in Humans." *Journal of Clinical Investigation*. 123.8 (2013): 3404–408. Web.

Zhao, Emmeline. "Best Education in The World: Finland, South Korea Top Country Rankings, U.S. Rated Average." *The Huffington Post*. 27 November 2012. Web. 7 June 2016.

Zuckerman, Marvin. *Sensation Seeking and Risky Behavior*. Washington, DC: American Psychological Association, 2007. Print.

About the Author

Erik Shonstrom is the author of *Wild Curiosity: How to Unleash Creativity and Encourage Lifelong Wondering* and is a professor of rhetoric and interdisciplinary studies at Champlain College. Erik has spent twenty years in education, much of it either exploring the outdoors or escaping the indoors. He lives in Vermont with his family.

CPSIA information can be obtained
at www.ICGtesting.com
Printed in the USA
BVOW08*1340271017
498558BV00002B/7/P

9 781475 825909